The Pharmacy Technician's Pocket Drug Reference

The Pharmacy Technician's Pocket Drug Reference

8th Edition

Theresa McEvoy, PharmD, BCPS
Clinical Pharmacy Specialist
Jonathan M. Wainwright Memorial VA Medical Center
Walla Walla, Washington

American Pharmacists Association
Improving medication use. Advancing patient care.

APhA   Washington, D.C.

Editor: Linda Young
Layout and Graphics: Michele Danoff, Graphics By Design
Cover Design: Mariam Safi and Scott Neitzke, APhA Creative Services

© 2015 by the American Pharmacists Association
Published by the American Pharmacists Association
2215 Constitution Avenue, N.W., Washington, DC 20037-2985
www.pharmacist.com   www.pharmacylibrary.com

APhA was founded in 1852 as the American Pharmaceutical Association.

To comment on this book via e-mail, send your message to the publisher at
aphabooks@aphanet.org.

Library of Congress Cataloging-in-Publication Data

McEvoy, Theresa, author.
    The pharmacy technician's pocket drug reference/Theresa McEvoy.—8th ed.
        p. ; cm.
    Preceeded by: Pharmacy technician's pocket drug reference/Joyce A.
Generali. c2013.
    Includes index.
    ISBN 978-1-58212-226-7
    I. Generali, Joyce A. Pharmacy technician's pocket drug reference. Preceded
by (work): II. American Pharmacists Association, publisher. III. Title.
    [DNLM: 1. Pharmaceutical Preparations—administration & dosage—
Handbooks. 2. Pharmacists' Aides—Handbooks. QV 735]
    RS122.95

    615.1—dc23

                            2014041876

How to Order This Book

Online: www.pharmacist.com/shop
By phone: 800-878-0729 (770-280-0085 from outside the United States)
VISA®, MasterCard®, and American Express® cards accepted

CONTENTS

Because the Food and Drug Administration (FDA) approves approximately 20 to 30 new chemical entities annually, keeping current with new drug products is a continuing concern for pharmacy technicians as well as pharmacists. *The Pharmacy Technician's Pocket Drug Reference* is the first drug information reference designed especially to help pharmacy technicians quickly identify drug products, their uses, and their dosage forms. The drugs included are categorized by generic names, trade names, therapeutic drug classes, general FDA-approved therapeutic uses, and commercially available dosage forms.

Kept concise for quick and easy access, the book can be used at work or during study for examination. When more in-depth drug information is required, referral to other drug information resources and consultation with the supervising pharmacist are always recommended.

Although several brand names are listed for most generic drugs, please note that this is for identification purposes only and does not infer or imply therapeutic or generic equivalency. In addition, all dosage forms may not be available for every trade name listed.

Special care has been taken to include the top 200 most commonly prescribed drugs. In addition, most drugs marketed since 1997 have been included in an attempt to create a resource that is useful in the practice setting.

Note that the information on most injectable formulations is presented in final dose amounts of the container (e.g., syringe, vial, ampul) and not as the concentration of the drug. Amounts provided for injectable formulations are not to be construed as appropriate doses. Some amounts are larger than typical doses because the container is a multidose vial. This resource is not intended as a dosing guide; an appropriate resource should be used in making patient care decisions. The inclusion of more than one brand name and product description in the same monograph does not imply therapeutic equivalence.

I hope this is a useful addition to your library and optimizes the efficient and safe practice of pharmacy.

Theresa McEvoy, Pharm D, BCPS
October 2014

ABACAVIR
a BAK a veer
TRADE NAME(S):
Ziagen
THERAPEUTIC CLASS:
Antiviral
GENERAL USES:
HIV infection
DOSAGE FORMS:
Tablets: 300 mg; Solution:
20 mg/mL

**ABACAVIR/
DOLUTEGRAVIR/
LAMIVUDINE**
a BAK a veer/DOE loo TEG
ra veer/la MI vyoo deen
TRADE NAME(S):
Triumeq
THERAPEUTIC CLASS:
Antiviral
GENERAL USES:
HIV infection
DOSAGE FORMS:
Tablets: 600 mg/50 mg/300
mg

ABACAVIR/LAMIVUDINE
a BAK a veer/la MI vyoo
deen
TRADE NAME(S):
Epzicom
THERAPEUTIC CLASS:
Antiviral
GENERAL USES:
HIV infection
DOSAGE FORMS:
Tablets: 600 mg/300 mg

**ABACAVIR/LAMIVUDINE/
ZIDOVUDINE**
a BAK a veer/la MI vyoo
deen/zye DOE vyoo deen
TRADE NAME(S):
Trizivir
THERAPEUTIC CLASS:
Antiviral
GENERAL USES:
HIV infection
DOSAGE FORMS:
Tablets: 300 mg/150 mg/
300 mg

ABATACEPT
ab a TA sept
TRADE NAME(S):
Orencia
THERAPEUTIC CLASS:
Antirheumatic
GENERAL USES:
Rheumatoid arthritis
DOSAGE FORMS:
Injection: 250 mg

ABIRATERONE ACETATE
A bir A ter one AS e tate
TRADE NAME(S):
Zytiga
THERAPEUTIC CLASS:
Antineoplastic
GENERAL USES:
Prostate cancer
DOSAGE FORMS:
Tablets: 250 mg

ABOBOTULINUMTOXINA
AY boe BOT yoo li num
TOKS in AY
TRADE NAME(S):
    Dysport
THERAPEUTIC CLASS:
    Toxoid
GENERAL USES:
    Cervical dystonia, facial
    wrinkles
DOSAGE FORMS:
    Injection: 300 units,
    500 units

**ACAMPROSATE
CALCIUM**
ay CAM pro sate
TRADE NAME(S):
    Campral
THERAPEUTIC CLASS:
    Antialcoholism agent
GENERAL USES:
    Alcohol dependence
DOSAGE FORMS:
    Delayed-release tablets:
    333 mg

ACARBOSE
AY car bose
TRADE NAME(S):
    Precose
THERAPEUTIC CLASS:
    Antidiabetic
GENERAL USES:
    Diabetes (type 2)
DOSAGE FORMS:
    Tablets: 25 mg, 50 mg,
    100 mg

ACEBUTOLOL
a se BYOO toe lole
TRADE NAME(S):
    Sectral
THERAPEUTIC CLASS:
    Antihypertensive,
    antiarrhythmic
GENERAL USES:
    Hypertension, arrhythmias
DOSAGE FORMS:
    Capsules: 200 mg,
    400 mg

ACETAMINOPHEN
a seet a MIN oh fen
TRADE NAME(S):
    Tylenol, Tempra, Aceta,
    Ofirmev, many others
THERAPEUTIC CLASS:
    Analgesic,
    antipyretic
GENERAL USES:
    Pain, fever
DOSAGE FORMS:
    Tablets: 160 mg,
    325 mg, 650 mg;
    Chewable tablets: 80 mg;
    Caplets: 160 mg;
    Capsules: 325 mg;
    Drops: 80 mg/0.8 mL;
    Also Elixir, Liquid,
    and Solution;
    Injection: 1000 mg

ACETOHEXAMIDE
a set oh HEKS a mide
TRADE NAME(S):
    Dymelor

THERAPEUTIC CLASS:
Antidiabetic
GENERAL USES:
Diabetes (type 2)
DOSAGE FORMS:
Tablets: 250 mg, 500 mg

ACETYLCYSTEINE
a se teel SIS teen
TRADE NAME(S):
Acetadote, Mucomyst
THERAPEUTIC CLASS:
Antidote
GENERAL USES:
Acetaminophen overdose
DOSAGE FORMS:
Injection: 20%;
Solution: 10%, 20%

ACITRETIN
a si TRE tin
TRADE NAME(S):
Soriatane
THERAPEUTIC CLASS:
Retinoid
GENERAL USES:
Psoriasis
DOSAGE FORMS:
Capsules: 10 mg, 25 mg

ACLIDINIUM BROMIDE
a kli DIN ee um
TRADE NAME(S):
Tudorza Pressair
THERAPEUTIC CLASS:
Respiratory agent
GENERAL USES:
Bronchospasm in COPD,
chronic bronchitis,
emphysema
DOSAGE FORMS:
Inhalation: 400 mcg/
actuation

ACYCLOVIR
ay SYE kloe veer
TRADE NAME(S):
Sitavig, Zovirax
THERAPEUTIC CLASS:
Antiviral
GENERAL USES:
Herpes, shingles,
chickenpox
DOSAGE FORMS:
Tablets: 400 mg,
800 mg; Buccal tablet:
50 mg; Capsules:
200 mg; Suspension:
200 mg/5 mL; Cream
and Ointment: 5%;
Injection: 500 mg, 1 g

ACYCLOVIR/ HYDROCORTISONE (TOPICAL)
ay SYE kloe veer/hye droe
KOR ti sone
TRADE NAME(S):
Xerese
THERAPEUTIC CLASS:
Antiviral/anti-
inflammatory (topical)
GENERAL USES:
Cold sores
DOSAGE FORMS:
Cream: 5%/1%

ADALIMUMAB
a da LIM yoo mab
Trade Name(s):
Humira
Therapeutic Class:
Monoclonal antibody
General Uses:
Rheumatoid arthritis,
ankylosing spondylitis,
inflammatory bowel disease
Dosage Forms:
Injection: 40 mg

ADAPALENE
a DAP a leen
Trade Name(s):
Differin
Therapeutic Class:
Retinoid (topical)
General Uses:
Acne vulgaris
Dosage Forms:
Topical gel, Cream,
Solution: 0.1%, 0.3%;
Topical lotion: 0.1%

ADAPALENE/BENZOYL PEROXIDE
a DAP a leen/BEN zoyl per
OKS ide
Trade Name(s):
Epiduo
Therapeutic Class:
Retinoid/anti-infective
(topical)
General Uses:
Acne
Dosage Forms:
Gel: 0.1%/2.5%

ADEFOVIR DIPIVOXIL
a DEF o veer dye pi
VOKS il
Trade Name(s):
Hepsera
Therapeutic Class:
Antiviral
General Uses:
Chronic hepatitis B
Dosage Forms:
Tablets: 10 mg

ADO-TRASTUZUMAB EMTANSINE
A doe tras TOOZ yoo mab
em TAN seen
Trade Name(s):
Kadcyla
Therapeutic Class:
Antineoplastic
General Uses:
Breast cancer
Dosage Forms:
Injection: 100 mg, 160 mg

AFATINIB DIMALEATE
a FAT i nib
Trade Name(s):
Gilotrif
Therapeutic Class:
Antineoplastic
General Uses:
Non—small-cell lung
cancer

DOSAGE FORMS:
Tablets: 20 mg, 30 mg,
40 mg

AFLIBERCEPT
a FLIB er cept
TRADE NAME(S):
Eylea
THERAPEUTIC CLASS:
Ocular agent
GENERAL USES:
Macular degeneration
(wet), macular edema
DOSAGE FORMS:
Injection: 40 mg/mL

AGALSIDASE BETA
ay GAL si days
TRADE NAME(S):
Fabrazyme
THERAPEUTIC CLASS:
Enzyme
GENERAL USES:
Fabry's disease
DOSAGE FORMS:
Injection: 5 mg, 35 mg

ALBIGLUTIDE
AL bi GLOO tide
TRADE NAME(S):
Tanzeum
THERAPEUTIC CLASS:
Antidiabetic
GENERAL USES:
Diabetes (type 2)
DOSAGE FORMS:
Injection: 30 mg, 50 mg

ALBUTEROL
al BYOO ter ole
TRADE NAME(S):
ProAir HFA, Proventil,
Proventil HFA,
Ventolin HFA
THERAPEUTIC CLASS:
Bronchodilator
GENERAL USES:
Bronchospasm
DOSAGE FORMS:
Tablets: 2 mg, 4 mg;
Extended-release
tablets: 4 mg, 8 mg;
Syrup: 2 mg/5 mL;
Aerosol: 90 mcg/
inhalation; Inhalation
solution: 0.021%,
0.042%, 0.083%, 0.5%

ALCAFTADINE (OCULAR)
al KAF ta deen
TRADE NAME(S):
Lastacaft
THERAPEUTIC CLASS:
Ocular agent
(antihistamine)
GENERAL USES:
Allergic conjunctivitis
DOSAGE FORMS:
Ophthalmic solution:
0.25%

ALCLOMETASONE
al kloe MET a sone
TRADE NAME(S):
Aclovate

THERAPEUTIC CLASS:
Corticosteroid
GENERAL USES:
Various skin conditions
DOSAGE FORMS:
Ointment and Cream:
0.05%

ALEFACEPT
a LE fa sept
TRADE NAME(S):
Amevive
THERAPEUTIC CLASS:
Monoclonal antibody
GENERAL USES:
Plaque psoriasis
DOSAGE FORMS:
Injection: 15 mg

ALEMTUZUMAB
ay lem TU zoo mab
TRADE NAME(S):
Campath
THERAPEUTIC CLASS:
Monoclonal antibody
GENERAL USES:
Refractory leukemia
DOSAGE FORMS:
Injection: 30 mg

ALENDRONATE
a LEN droe nate
TRADE NAME(S):
Fosamax, Binosto
THERAPEUTIC CLASS:
Bisphosphonate

GENERAL USES:
Osteoporosis, Paget's
disease
DOSAGE FORMS:
Tablets: 5 mg, 10 mg,
35 mg, 40 mg, 70 mg;
Effervescent tablets:
70 mg; Oral solution:
70 mg/75 mL

ALENDRONATE/
CHOLECALCIFEROL
a LEN droe nate/kole eh kal
SI fer ole
TRADE NAME(S):
Fosamax Plus D
THERAPEUTIC CLASS:
Bisphosphonate/
vitamin
GENERAL USES:
Osteoporosis
DOSAGE FORMS:
Tablets: 70 mg/
2800 international units
(IU), 70 mg/5600 IU

ALFUZOSIN
al FYOO zoe sin
TRADE NAME(S):
Uroxatral
THERAPEUTIC CLASS:
Urologic agent
GENERAL USES:
BPH
DOSAGE FORMS:
Extended-release tablets:
10 mg

ALGLUCOSIDASE ALFA
al gloo KOSE i dase AL fa
TRADE NAME(S):
Lumizyme, Myozyme
THERAPEUTIC CLASS:
Enzyme
GENERAL USES:
Pompe disease
DOSAGE FORMS:
Injection: 50 mg

ALISKIREN
a lis KYE ren
TRADE NAME(S):
Tekturna
THERAPEUTIC CLASS:
Antihypertensive
GENERAL USES:
Hypertension
DOSAGE FORMS:
Tablets: 150 mg, 300 mg

ALISKIREN/AMLODIPINE
a lis KYE ren/am LOE di
peen
TRADE NAME(S):
Tekamlo
THERAPEUTIC CLASS:
Antihypertensive
GENERAL USES:
Hypertension
DOSAGE FORMS:
Tablets: 150 mg/5 mg,
150 mg/10 mg, 300 mg/
5 mg, 300 mg/10 mg

ALISKIREN/HCTZ
a lis KYE ren/hye droe klor
oh THYE a zide
TRADE NAME(S):
Tekturna HCT
THERAPEUTIC CLASS:
Antihypertensive/
diuretic
GENERAL USES:
Hypertension
DOSAGE FORMS:
Tablets: 150 mg/12.5 mg,
150 mg/25 mg, 300 mg/
12.5 mg, 300 mg/25 mg

ALISKIREN/VALSARTAN
a lis KYE ren/val SAR tan
TRADE NAME(S):
Valturna
THERAPEUTIC CLASS:
Antihypertensive
GENERAL USES:
Hypertension
DOSAGE FORMS:
Tablets: 150 mg/160 mg,
300 mg/320 mg

ALITRETINOIN
a li TRET i noyn
TRADE NAME(S):
Panretin
THERAPEUTIC CLASS:
Retinoid (topical)
GENERAL USES:
Kaposi's sarcoma
cutaneous lesions
DOSAGE FORMS:
Topical gel: 0.1%

ALLOPURINOL
al oh PURE i nole
TRADE NAME(S):
  Zyloprim
THERAPEUTIC CLASS:
  Gout agent
GENERAL USES:
  Gout, increased uric
  acid conditions, calcium
  stones
DOSAGE FORMS:
  Tablets: 100 mg, 300 mg;
  Injection: 500 mg

ALMOTRIPTAN
al moh TRIP tan
TRADE NAME(S):
  Axert
THERAPEUTIC CLASS:
  Antimigraine agent
GENERAL USES:
  Migraine treatment
DOSAGE FORMS:
  Tablets: 6.25 mg, 12.5 mg

ALOGLIPTIN
AL oh GLIP tin
TRADE NAME(S):
  Nesina
THERAPEUTIC CLASS:
  Antidiabetic
GENERAL USES:
  Diabetes (type 2)
DOSAGE FORMS:
  Tablets: 6.25 mg,
  12.5 mg, 25 mg

**ALOGLIPTIN/
METFORMIN**
AL oh GLIP tin/MET for min
TRADE NAME(S):
  Kazano
THERAPEUTIC CLASS:
  Antidiabetic
GENERAL USES:
  Diabetes (type 2)
DOSAGE FORMS:
  Tablets: 12.5 mg/500 mg,
  12.5 mg/1000 mg

**ALOGLIPTIN/
PIOGLITAZONE**
AL oh GLIP tin/pye oh GLI
ta zone
TRADE NAME(S):
  Oseni
THERAPEUTIC CLASS:
  Antidiabetic
GENERAL USES:
  Diabetes (type 2)
DOSAGE FORMS:
  Tablets: 12.5 mg/15 mg,
  12.5 mg/30 mg, 12.5 mg/
  45 mg, 25 mg/15 mg,
  25 mg/30 mg, 25 mg/45 mg

ALOSETRON
al OH seh trahn
TRADE NAME(S):
  Lotronex
THERAPEUTIC CLASS:
  GI agent
GENERAL USES:
  Irritable bowel syndrome
  (women)

DOSAGE FORMS:
Tablets: 0.5 mg, 1 mg

ALPRAZOLAM
al PRAY zoe lam
TRADE NAME(S):
Xanax, Xanax XR,
Alprazolam Intensol,
Niravam
THERAPEUTIC CLASS:
Antianxiety agent
GENERAL USES:
Anxiety, panic disorder
DOSAGE FORMS:
Tablets: 0.25 mg,
0.5 mg, 1 mg, 2 mg;
Solution: 1 mg/mL;
Extended-release tablets:
0.5 mg, 1 mg, 2 mg, 3 mg;
Orally disintegrating
tablets: 0.25 mg, 0.5 mg,
1 mg, 2 mg

ALTEPLASE
AL te plase
TRADE NAME(S):
Activase,
Cathflo Activase
THERAPEUTIC CLASS:
Thrombolytic agent
GENERAL USES:
Dissolves blood clots in
MI, stroke, pulmonary
embolism, catheter
occlusion
DOSAGE FORMS:
Injection: 2 mg, 50 mg,
100 mg

ALVIMOPAN
al vi MOE pan
TRADE NAME(S):
Entereg
THERAPEUTIC CLASS:
GI agent
GENERAL USES:
Postoperative ileus
DOSAGE FORMS:
Capsules: 12 mg

AMANTADINE
a MAN ta deen
TRADE NAME(S):
Symmetrel
THERAPEUTIC CLASS:
Antiparkinson agent
GENERAL USES:
Parkinson's disease,
drug-induced
extrapyramidal
disorders
DOSAGE FORMS:
Tablets and Capsules:
100 mg; Syrup: 50 mg/
5 mL

AMBRISENTAN
am bree SEN tan
TRADE NAME(S):
Letairis
THERAPEUTIC CLASS:
Antihypertensive
GENERAL USES:
Pulmonary hypertension
DOSAGE FORMS:
Tablets: 5 mg, 10 mg

AMCINONIDE
am SIN oh nide
TRADE NAME(S):
Cyclocort
THERAPEUTIC CLASS:
Corticosteroid (topical)
GENERAL USES:
Various skin conditions
DOSAGE FORMS:
Ointment, Cream, and
Lotion: 0.1%

AMIKACIN
am i KAY sin
TRADE NAME(S):
Amikin
THERAPEUTIC CLASS:
Anti-infective
GENERAL USES:
Bacterial infections
DOSAGE FORMS:
Injection: 100 mg,
200 mg, 500 mg, 1 g

AMILORIDE
a MIL oh ride
TRADE NAME(S):
Midamor
THERAPEUTIC CLASS:
Diuretic
GENERAL USES:
CHF-related edema,
hypertension
DOSAGE FORMS:
Tablets: 5 mg

AMINOCAPROIC ACID
a mee noe ka PROE ik
TRADE NAME(S):
Amicar
THERAPEUTIC CLASS:
Hemostatic
GENERAL USES:
Excessive bleeding
DOSAGE FORMS:
Tablets: 500 mg; Syrup:
250 mg/mL

AMINOLEVULINIC ACID
a MEE noh lev yoo lin ik
TRADE NAME(S):
Levulan Kerastick
THERAPEUTIC CLASS:
Skin agent (topical)
GENERAL USES:
Precancerous skin lesions
on face or scalp
DOSAGE FORMS:
Topical solution: 20%

AMINOPHYLLINE
am in OFF i lin
TRADE NAME(S)
Phyllocontin
THERAPEUTIC CLASS:
Bronchodilator
GENERAL USES:
Asthma
DOSAGE FORMS:
(equivalent amount of
theophylline):
Tablets: 100 mg (79 mg),
200 mg (158 mg);

Controlled-release tablets:
225 mg (178 mg);
Oral liquid: 105 mg/5 mL
(90 mg/5 mL);
Injection: 250 mg
(197 mg), 500 mg
(394 mg)

AMIODARONE
a MEE oh da rone
TRADE NAME(S):
Cordarone, Cordarone IV,
Pacerone
THERAPEUTIC CLASS:
Antiarrhythmic
GENERAL USES:
Ventricular
arrhythmias and
fibrillation
DOSAGE FORMS:
Tablets: 100 mg, 200 mg,
300 mg, 400 mg;
Injection: 150 mg

AMITRIPTYLINE
a mee TRIP ti leen
TRADE NAME(S):
Elavil
THERAPEUTIC CLASS:
Antidepressant
GENERAL USES:
Depression
DOSAGE FORMS:
Tablets: 10 mg, 25 mg,
50 mg, 75 mg, 100 mg,
150 mg

AMLODIPINE
am LOE di peen
TRADE NAME(S):
Norvasc
THERAPEUTIC CLASS:
Antihypertensive,
antianginal
GENERAL USES:
Angina, hypertension
DOSAGE FORMS:
Tablets: 2.5 mg, 5 mg,
10 mg

AMLODIPINE/ATORVASTATIN
am LOE di peen/a TORE va
sta tin
TRADE NAME(S):
Caduet
THERAPEUTIC CLASS:
Antihypertensive/
antilipemic
GENERAL USES:
Hypertension, angina,
lipid disorders
DOSAGE FORMS:
Tablets: 2.5 mg/10 mg,
5 mg/10 mg, 10 mg/
10 mg, 2.5 mg/20 mg,
5 mg/20 mg, 10 mg/
20 mg, 2.5 mg/40 mg,
5 mg/40 mg, 10 mg/
40 mg, 5 mg/80 mg,
10 mg/80 mg

AMLODIPINE/ BENAZEPRIL

am LOE di peen/ben AY ze pril

TRADE NAME(S):
Lotrel

THERAPEUTIC CLASS:
Antihypertensive/ diuretic

GENERAL USES:
CHF, hypertension

DOSAGE FORMS:
Tablets: 2.5 mg/10 mg, 5 mg/10 mg, 5 mg/20 mg, 5 mg/40 mg, 10 mg/ 20 mg, 10 mg/40 mg

AMLODIPINE/HCTZ/ OLMESARTAN

am LOE di peen/hye droe klor oh THYE a zide/ole me SAR tan

TRADE NAME(S):
Tribenzor

THERAPEUTIC CLASS:
Antihypertensive/diuretic

GENERAL USES:
Hypertension

DOSAGE FORMS:
Tablets: 5 mg/12.5 mg/ 20 mg, 5 mg/12.5 mg/ 40 mg, 5 mg/25 mg/ 40 mg, 10 mg/12.5 mg/ 40 mg, 10 mg/25 mg/ 40 mg

AMLODIPINE/HCTZ/ VALSARTAN

am LOE di peen/hye droe klor oh THYE a zide/val SAR tan

TRADE NAME(S):
Exforge HCT

THERAPEUTIC CLASS:
Antihypertensive/diuretic

GENERAL USES:
Hypertension

DOSAGE FORMS:
Tablets: 5 mg/12.5 mg/ 160 mg, 5 mg/25 mg/ 160 mg, 10 mg/12.5 mg/ 160 mg, 10 mg/25 mg/ 160 mg, 10 mg/25 mg/ 320 mg

AMLODIPINE/ OLMESARTAN

am LOE di peen/ole me SAR tan

TRADE NAME(S):
Azor

THERAPEUTIC CLASS:
Antihypertensive

GENERAL USES:
Hypertension

DOSAGE FORMS:
Tablets: 5 mg/20 mg, 5 mg/40 mg, 10 mg/ 20 mg, 10 mg/40 mg

AMLODIPINE/ TELMISARTAN

am LOE di peen/tel mi SAR tan

TRADE NAME(S):
Twynsta
THERAPEUTIC CLASS:
Antihypertensive
GENERAL USES:
Hypertension
DOSAGE FORMS:
Tablets: 5 mg/40 mg,
5 mg/80 mg, 10 mg/40 mg,
10 mg/80 mg

AMLODIPINE/ VALSARTAN
am LOE di peen/val SAR tan
TRADE NAME(S):
Exforge
THERAPEUTIC CLASS:
Antihypertensive
GENERAL USES:
Hypertension
DOSAGE FORMS:
Tablets: 5 mg/160 mg,
5 mg/320 mg, 10 mg/
160 mg, 10 mg/320 mg

AMOXAPINE
a MOKS a peen
TRADE NAME(S):
Asendin
THERAPEUTIC CLASS:
Antidepressant
GENERAL USES:
Depression
DOSAGE FORMS:
Tablets: 25 mg, 50 mg,
100 mg, 150 mg

AMOXICILLIN
a moks i SIL in
TRADE NAME(S):
Amoxicot, Amoxil, Moxatag,
Moxilin, Trimox, Wymox
THERAPEUTIC CLASS:
Anti-infective
GENERAL USES:
Bacterial infections
DOSAGE FORMS:
Chewable tablets: 125 mg,
200 mg, 250 mg, 400 mg;
Tablets: 500 mg, 875 mg;
Extended-release tablets:
775 mg; Capsules:
250 mg, 500 mg;
Suspension: 50 mg/mL,
125 mg/5 mL, 200 mg/
5 mL, 250 mg/5 mL,
400 mg/5 mL; Tablets for
oral suspension: 200 mg,
400 mg

AMOXICILLIN/ CLAVULANATE
a moks i SIL in/klav yoo
LAN ate
TRADE NAME(S):
Augmentin,
Augmentin ES,
Augmentin XR
THERAPEUTIC CLASS:
Anti-infective
GENERAL USES:
Bacterial infections
DOSAGE FORMS:
Tablets: 250 mg/125 mg,

500 mg/125 mg, 875 mg/
125 mg; Chewable tablets
and Suspension (per
5 mL): 125 mg/31.25 mg,
200 mg/28.5 mg,
250 mg/62.5 mg,
400 mg/57 mg; High-
dose suspension
(per 5 mL): 600 mg/
42.9 mg; Extended-
release tablets:
1000 mg/62.5 mg

**AMPHOTERICIN B
(ORAL)**
am foe TER i sin
TRADE NAME(S):
Fungizone
THERAPEUTIC CLASS:
Antifungal
GENERAL USES:
Oral fungal infection
(candidiasis)
DOSAGE FORMS:
Suspension: 100 mg/
mL; Cream, Lotion, and
Ointment: 3%

**AMPHOTERICIN B
DESOXYCHOLATE
(NONLIPID BASED)**
am foe TER i sin bee
des oks ee KOE late
TRADE NAME(S):
Fungizone, Amphocin
THERAPEUTIC CLASS:
Antifungal

GENERAL USES:
Systemic fungal infections
DOSAGE FORMS:
Injection: 50 mg

**AMPHOTERICIN B
(LIPID BASED)**
am foe TER i sin
TRADE NAME(S):
Abelcet, Amphotec,
AmBisome
THERAPEUTIC CLASS:
Antifungal
GENERAL USES:
Systemic fungal
infections
DOSAGE FORMS:
Injection: 50 mg, 100 mg

AMPICILLIN
am pi SIL in
TRADE NAME(S):
Principen, Omnipen,
Totacillin
THERAPEUTIC CLASS:
Anti-infective
GENERAL USES:
Bacterial infections
DOSAGE FORMS:
Capsules: 250 mg, 500 mg;
Suspension: 125 mg/
5 mL, 250 mg/5 mL;
Injection: 125 mg, 250 mg,
500 mg, 1 g, 2 g, 10 g

AMPICILLIN SODIUM/ SULBACTAM SODIUM
am pi SIL in/SUL bak tam
TRADE NAME(S):
Unasyn
THERAPEUTIC CLASS:
Anti-infective
GENERAL USES:
Bacterial infections
DOSAGE FORMS:
Injection: 1 g/0.5 g,
2 g/1 g, 10 g/5 g

ANAGRELIDE
an AG re lide
TRADE NAME(S):
Agrylin
THERAPEUTIC CLASS:
Antiplatelet agent
GENERAL USES:
Essential
thrombocytopenia
DOSAGE FORMS:
Capsules: 0.5 mg, 1 mg

ANAKINRA
an a KIN ra
TRADE NAME(S):
Kineret
THERAPEUTIC CLASS:
Biological
GENERAL USES:
Rheumatoid arthritis,
multisystem inflammatory
disease
DOSAGE FORMS:
Injection: 100 mg

ANASTROZOLE
an AS troe zole
TRADE NAME(S):
Arimidex
THERAPEUTIC CLASS:
Antineoplastic
GENERAL USES:
Breast cancer
DOSAGE FORMS:
Tablets: 1 mg

ANIDULAFUNGIN
ay nid yoo la FUN jin
TRADE NAME(S):
Eraxis
THERAPEUTIC CLASS:
Antifungal
GENERAL USES:
Candidemia, candidiasis
DOSAGE FORMS:
Injection: 50 mg, 100 mg

ANTHRALIN
AN thra lin
TRADE NAME(S):
Anthra-Derm,
Drithocreme
THERAPEUTIC CLASS:
Antipsoriatic (topical)
GENERAL USES:
Psoriasis
DOSAGE FORMS:
Ointment and Cream:
0.1%, 0.25%, 0.4%,
0.5%, 1%; Cream: 0.2%

ANTIHEMOPHILIC FACTOR (RECOMBINANT)
AN tee hee moe FIL ik

TRADE NAME(S):
Advate, Xyntha

THERAPEUTIC CLASS:
Hematological agent

GENERAL USES:
Prevent/control hemorrhage

DOSAGE FORMS:
Injection: 250 international units (IU), 500 IU, 1000 IU, 2000 IU, 3000 IU, 4000 IU

APIXABAN
a PIX a ban

TRADE NAME(S):
Eliquis

THERAPEUTIC CLASS:
Anticoagulant

GENERAL USES:
Reduce risk of stroke and clots

DOSAGE FORMS:
Tablets: 2.5 mg, 5 mg

APOMORPHINE
a poe MOR feen

TRADE NAME(S):
Apokyn

THERAPEUTIC CLASS:
Dopamine agonist

GENERAL USES:
Parkinson's disease

DOSAGE FORMS:
Injection: 20 mg, 30 mg

APRACLONIDINE
a pra KLOE ni deen

TRADE NAME(S):
Iopidine

THERAPEUTIC CLASS:
Ocular agent

GENERAL USES:
Decrease intraocular pressure

DOSAGE FORMS:
Ophthalmic solution: 0.5%, 1%

APREMILAST
a PRE mi last

TRADE NAME(S):
Otezla

THERAPEUTIC CLASS:
Musculoskeletal agent

GENERAL USES:
Psoriatic arthritis, psoriasis

DOSAGE FORMS:
Tablets: 10 mg, 20 mg, 30 mg

APREPITANT
ap RE pi tant

TRADE NAME(S):
Emend

THERAPEUTIC CLASS:
Antiemetic

GENERAL USES:
Chemotherapy-induced
or postoperative nausea/
vomiting
DOSAGE FORMS:
Capsules: 40 mg, 80 mg,
125 mg

ARFORMOTEROL
ar for MOE ter ol
TRADE NAME(S):
Brovana
THERAPEUTIC CLASS:
Bronchodilator
GENERAL USES:
COPD
DOSAGE FORMS:
Inhalation solution:
15 mcg/2 mL

ARGATROBAN
ar GA troh ban
TRADE NAME(S):
Acova
THERAPEUTIC CLASS:
Anticoagulant
GENERAL USES:
Anticoagulation in
hemodialysis or PCI
DOSAGE FORMS:
Injection: 250 mg

ARIPIPRAZOLE
ay ri PIP ray zole
TRADE NAME(S):
Abilify, Abilify Discmelt,
Abilify Maintena

THERAPEUTIC CLASS:
Antipsychotic
GENERAL USES:
Psychotic disorders
DOSAGE FORMS:
Tablets: 5 mg, 10 mg,
15 mg, 20 mg, 30 mg;
Oral solution: 1 mg/1 mL;
Orally disintegrating
tablets: 10 mg, 15 mg,
20 mg, 30 mg; Injection:
7.5 mg; Extended-release
injection: 300 mg, 400 mg

ARMODAFINIL
ar moe DAF in il
TRADE NAME(S):
Nuvigil
THERAPEUTIC CLASS:
Stimulant
GENERAL USES:
Excessive sleepiness,
narcolepsy, obstructive
sleep apnea
DOSAGE FORMS:
Tablets: 50 mg, 150 mg,
250 mg

ARSENIC TRIOXIDE
AR se nik tri OKS ide
TRADE NAME(S):
Trisenox
THERAPEUTIC CLASS:
Antineoplastic
GENERAL USES:
Acute promyelocytic
leukemia

DOSAGE FORMS:
    Injection: 10 mg

**ARTEMETHER/
LUMEFANTRINE**
ar TEM e ther/LOO me
FAN treen
TRADE NAME(S):
    Coartem
THERAPEUTIC CLASS:
    Anti-infective
GENERAL USES:
    Malaria
DOSAGE FORMS:
    Tablets: 20 mg/120 mg

**ASENAPINE MALEATE
(SUBLINGUAL)**
a SEN a peen
TRADE NAME(S):
    Saphris
THERAPEUTIC CLASS:
    Antipsychotic
GENERAL USES:
    Schizophrenia, mania
DOSAGE FORMS:
    Tablets: 5 mg, 10 mg

**ASPARAGINASE
*ERWINIA
CHRYSANTHEMI***
as PAR a jin ase
TRADE NAME(S):
    Erwinaze
THERAPEUTIC CLASS:
    Antineoplastic
GENERAL USES:
    ALL

DOSAGE FORMS:
    Injection: 10,000
    international units

ASPIRIN
AS pir in
TRADE NAME(S):
    Empirin, Zorprin, many
    others
THERAPEUTIC CLASS:
    Analgesic, antipyretic,
    anti-inflammatory
GENERAL USES:
    Pain, fever (adults),
    arthritis
DOSAGE FORMS:
    Tablets: 81 mg, 165 mg,
    325 mg, 500 mg,
    650 mg, 975 mg;
    Extended-release tablets:
    650 mg, 800 mg;
    Capsules: 325 mg

**ASPIRIN/
DIPYRIDAMOLE**
AS pir in/dye peer ID a mole
TRADE NAME(S):
    Aggrenox
THERAPEUTIC CLASS:
    Antithrombotic
GENERAL USES:
    Reduce stroke risk
DOSAGE FORMS:
    Capsules: 25 mg/
    200 mg

ATAZANAVIR SULFATE
at a za NA veer

Trade Name(s):
Reyataz

Therapeutic Class:
Antiviral

General Uses:
HIV infection

Dosage Forms:
Capsules: 100 mg,
150 mg, 200 mg, 300 mg;
Oral powder: 50 mg

ATENOLOL
a TEN oh lole

Trade Name(s):
Tenormin

Therapeutic Class:
Cardiac agent

General Uses:
Hypertension

Dosage Forms:
Tablets: 25 mg, 50 mg,
100 mg; Injection: 5 mg

ATENOLOL/
CHLORTHALIDONE
a TEN oh lole/klor THAL i
done

Trade Name(s):
Tenoretic

Therapeutic Class:
Antihypertensive/diuretic

General Uses:
Hypertension

Dosage Forms:
Tablets: 100 mg/25 mg,
50 mg/25 mg

ATOMOXETINE
AT oh moks e teen

Trade Name(s):
Strattera

Therapeutic Class:
Nonstimulant agent

General Uses:
ADHD

Dosage Forms:
Capsules: 10 mg, 18 mg,
25 mg, 40 mg, 60 mg,
80 mg, 100 mg

ATORVASTATIN
a TORE va sta tin

Trade Name(s):
Lipitor

Therapeutic Class:
Antilipemic

General Uses:
Hyperlipidemia,
hypertriglyceridemia,
reduce stroke or MI risk

Dosage Forms:
Tablets: 10 mg, 20 mg,
40 mg, 80 mg

ATOVAQUONE/
PROGUANIL
a TOE va kwone/pro
GWA nil

Trade Name(s):
Malarone,
Malarone-Pediatric

Therapeutic Class:
Antimalarial

General Uses:
Malaria treatment and

prevention
DOSAGE FORMS:
Tablets: 250 mg/100 mg,
62.5 mg/25 mg

ATROPINE
A troe peen
TRADE NAME(S):
Isopto Atropine
THERAPEUTIC CLASS:
Ocular agent
GENERAL USES:
Pupil dilation
DOSAGE FORMS:
Ophthalmic solution:
0.5%, 1%, 2%;
Ophthalmic ointment: 1%

AURANOFIN
au RANE oh fin
TRADE NAME(S):
Ridaura
THERAPEUTIC CLASS:
Antirheumatic agent
GENERAL USES:
Rheumatoid arthritis
DOSAGE FORMS:
Capsules: 3 mg

AVANAFIL
a VAN a fil
TRADE NAME(S):
Stendra
THERAPEUTIC CLASS:
Impotence agent
GENERAL USES:
Erectile dysfunction

DOSAGE FORMS:
Tablets: 50 mg, 100 mg,
200 mg

AXITINIB
aks I ti nib
TRADE NAME(S):
Inlyta
THERAPEUTIC CLASS:
Antineoplastic
GENERAL USES:
Kidney cancer
DOSAGE FORMS:
Tablets: 1 mg, 5 mg

AZACITIDINE
ay za SYE ti deen
TRADE NAME(S):
Vidaza
THERAPEUTIC CLASS:
Antineoplastic
GENERAL USES:
Myelodysplastic
syndrome
DOSAGE FORMS:
Injection: 100 mg

AZELASTINE (NASAL)
a ZEL as teen
TRADE NAME(S):
Astelin, Astepro
THERAPEUTIC CLASS:
Antihistamine
GENERAL USES:
Allergies
DOSAGE FORMS:
Nasal spray: 125 mcg/
spray, 137 mcg/spray

AZELASTINE (OCULAR)
a ZEL as teen
TRADE NAME(S):
Optivar
THERAPEUTIC CLASS:
Ocular agent
(antihistamine)
GENERAL USES:
Allergic conjunctivitis
DOSAGE FORMS:
Ophthalmic solution:
0.05%

**AZELASTINE/
FLUTICASONE (NASAL)**
a ZEL as teen/floo TIK a sone
TRADE NAME(S):
Dymista
THERAPEUTIC CLASS:
Antihistamine/
corticosteroid
GENERAL USES:
Seasonal allergies
DOSAGE FORMS:
Nasal spray: 137 mcg/
50 mcg per spray

**AZILSARTAN
MEDOXOMIL**
AY zil SAR tan
me DOKS oh mil
TRADE NAME(S):
Edarbi
THERAPEUTIC CLASS:
Antihypertensive
GENERAL USES:
Hypertension

DOSAGE FORMS:
Tablets: 40 mg, 80 mg

**AZILSARTAN
MEDOXOMIL/
CHLORTHALIDONE**
AY zil SAR tan me DOKS oh
mil/klor THAL i done
TRADE NAME(S):
Edarbyclor
THERAPEUTIC CLASS:
Antihypertensive/diuretic
GENERAL USES:
Hypertension
DOSAGE FORMS:
Tablets: 40 mg/12.5 mg,
40 mg/25 mg

AZITHROMYCIN
az ith roe MYE sin
TRADE NAME(S):
Zithromax, Zmax
THERAPEUTIC CLASS:
Anti-infective
GENERAL USES:
Bacterial infections
DOSAGE FORMS:
Tablets: 250 mg, 500 mg,
600 mg; Suspension:
100 mg/5 mL, 200 mg/
5 mL; Injection: 500 mg

**AZITHROMYCIN
(OCULAR)**
az ith roe MYE sin
TRADE NAME(S):
AzaSite

Therapeutic Class:
Anti-infective (ocular)
General Uses:
Bacterial conjunctivitis
Dosage Forms:
Ophthalmic solution: 1%

AZTREONAM
AZ tree oh nam
Trade Name(s):
Azactam
Therapeutic Class:
Anti-infective
General Uses:
Bacterial infections
Dosage Forms:
Injection: 500 mg,
1 g, 2 g

**AZTREONAM
(INHALATION)**
AZ tree oh nam
Trade Name(s):
Cayston
Therapeutic Class:
Anti-infective
General Uses:
Bacterial lung infections
Dosage Forms:
Solution for inhalation:
75 mg

BACITRACIN
bas i TRAY sin
Trade Name(s):
AK-Tracin

Therapeutic Class:
Ocular agent
(anti-infective)
General Uses:
Ocular infections
Dosage Forms:
Ophthalmic ointment:
500 units/g

BACLOFEN
BAK loe fen
Trade Name(s):
Gablofen, Lioresal,
Lioresal Intrathecal
Therapeutic Class:
Skeletal muscle relaxant
General Uses:
Spasticity
Dosage Forms:
Tablets: 10 mg, 20 mg;
Injection: 0.05 mg,
0.5 mg, 2 mg, 10 mg,
20 mg, 40 mg

BALSALAZIDE
bal SAL a zide
Trade Name(s):
Colazal, Giazo
Therapeutic Class:
GI agent
General Uses:
Ulcerative colitis
Dosage Forms:
Capsules: 750 mg;
Tablets: 1.1 g

BAZEDOXIFENE/ CONJUGATED ESTROGENS

BA ze DOKS i feen/KON joo GAY ted ES troe jens

TRADE NAME(S):
Duavee

THERAPEUTIC CLASS:
Hormone (estrogen), antiestrogen

GENERAL USES:
Vasomotor symptoms of menopause, prevent postmenopausal osteoporosis

DOSAGE FORMS:
Tablets: 20 mg/0.45 mg

BECAPLERMIN

be KAP ler min

TRADE NAME(S):
Regranex

THERAPEUTIC CLASS:
Wound healer (topical)

GENERAL USES:
Diabetic neuropathic ulcers

DOSAGE FORMS:
Topical gel: 0.01%

BECLOMETHASONE (INHALED)

be kloe METH a sone

TRADE NAME(S):
Vanceril, Beclovent, Qvar

THERAPEUTIC CLASS:
Corticosteroid (inhaler)

GENERAL USES:
Asthma (chronic)

DOSAGE FORMS:
Inhaler:
40 mcg/inhalation,
42 mcg/inhalation,
80 mcg/inhalation,
84 mcg/inhalation

BECLOMETHASONE (NASAL)

be kloe METH a sone

TRADE NAME(S):
Beconase, Vancenase, Beconase AQ, QNASL, Vancenase AQ

THERAPEUTIC CLASS:
Corticosteroid (nasal)

GENERAL USES:
Allergies

DOSAGE FORMS:
Nasal spray: 0.042%, 0.084%; Nasal aerosol: 0.08%

BEDAQUILINE

bed AK wi leen

TRADE NAME(S):
Sirturo

THERAPEUTIC CLASS:
Antituberculosis agent

GENERAL USES:
Multi-drug resistant tuberculosis

DOSAGE FORMS:
Tablets: 100 mg

BELATACEPT
bel AT a sept
TRADE NAME(S):
Nulojix
THERAPEUTIC CLASS:
Immunosuppressant
GENERAL USES:
Prevent organ rejection
DOSAGE FORMS:
Injection: 250 mg

BELIMUMAB
be LIM yoo mab
TRADE NAME(S):
Benlysta
THERAPEUTIC CLASS:
Monoclonal antibody
GENERAL USES:
SLE
DOSAGE FORMS:
Injection: 120 mg, 400 mg

BELINOSTAT
be LIN oh stat
TRADE NAME(S):
Beleodaq
THERAPEUTIC CLASS:
Antineoplastic
GENERAL USES:
Peripheral T-cell
lymphoma
DOSAGE FORMS:
Injection: 500 mg

BENAZEPRIL
ben AY ze pril
TRADE NAME(S):
Lotensin

THERAPEUTIC CLASS:
Antihypertensive
GENERAL USES:
Hypertension
DOSAGE FORMS:
Tablets: 5 mg, 10 mg,
20 mg, 40 mg

BENAZEPRIL/HCTZ
ben AY ze pril/hye droe klor
oh THYE a zide
TRADE NAME(S):
Lotensin HCT
THERAPEUTIC CLASS:
Antihypertensive/
diuretic
GENERAL USES:
Hypertension
DOSAGE FORMS:
Tablets: 5 mg/6.25 mg,
10 mg/12.5 mg, 20 mg/
12.5 mg, 20 mg/25 mg

BENDAMUSTINE
ben da MUS teen
TRADE NAME(S):
Treanda
THERAPEUTIC CLASS:
Antineoplastic
GENERAL USES:
CLL, non-Hodgkin's
lymphoma
DOSAGE FORMS:
Injection: 100 mg

BENZONATATE
ben ZOE na tate
TRADE NAME(S):
Tessalon Perles

THERAPEUTIC CLASS:
Nonnarcotic cough
suppressant
GENERAL USES:
Relief of cough
DOSAGE FORMS:
Capsules: 100 mg

BENZOYL PEROXIDE
BEN zoyl per OKS ide
TRADE NAME(S):
Benzac, PanOxyl, Persa-
Gel, many others
THERAPEUTIC CLASS:
Anti-infective (topical)
GENERAL USES:
Acne
DOSAGE FORMS:
Liquid, Lotion, Cream,
Gel: 2.5%, 5%, 10%

BENZOYL PEROXIDE/ CLINDAMYCIN (TOPICAL)
BEN zoyl per OKS ide/klin
da MYE sin
TRADE NAME(S):
BenzaClin, Duac
THERAPEUTIC CLASS:
Anti-infective (topical)
GENERAL USES:
Acne
DOSAGE FORMS:
Gel: 5%/1%

BENZTROPINE
BENZ troe peen
TRADE NAME(S):
Cogentin

THERAPEUTIC CLASS:
Antiparkinson agent
GENERAL USES:
Parkinson's disease,
drug-induced
extrapyramidal disorders
DOSAGE FORMS:
Tablets: 0.5 mg, 1 mg,
2 mg

BENZYL ALCOHOL
BEN zil AL ka hol
TRADE NAME(S):
Ulesfia
THERAPEUTIC CLASS:
Pediculicide (topical)
GENERAL USES:
Head lice
DOSAGE FORMS:
Lotion: 5%

BEPOTASTINE BESILATE (OCULAR)
bep oh TAS teen
TRADE NAME(S):
Bepreve
THERAPEUTIC CLASS:
Ocular agent
(antihistamine)
GENERAL USES:
Allergic conjunctivitis
DOSAGE FORMS:
Ophthalmic solution: 1.5%

BEPRIDIL
BE pri dil
TRADE NAME(S):
Vascor

THERAPEUTIC CLASS:
Antianginal

GENERAL USES:
Angina

DOSAGE FORMS:
Tablets: 200 mg, 300 mg, 400 mg

BESIFLOXACIN HCL (OCULAR)
BE si FLOKS a sin

TRADE NAME(S):
Besivance

THERAPEUTIC CLASS:
Ocular agent (anti-infective)

GENERAL USES:
Ocular infections

DOSAGE FORMS:
Ophthalmic suspension: 0.6%

BETAMETHASONE DIPROPIONATE
bay ta METH a sone

TRADE NAME(S):
Diprosone, Alphatrex, Maxivate

THERAPEUTIC CLASS:
Corticosteroid (topical)

GENERAL USES:
Various skin conditions

DOSAGE FORMS:
Ointment, Cream, and Lotion: 0.05%; Aerosol: 0.1%

BETAMETHASONE VALERATE
bay ta METH a sone

TRADE NAME(S):
Betatrex, Valisone

THERAPEUTIC CLASS:
Corticosteroid (topical)

GENERAL USES:
Various skin conditions

DOSAGE FORMS:
Ointment, Cream, and Lotion: 0.1%; Cream: 0.01%, 0.05%

BETAXOLOL (OCULAR)
be TAKS oh lol

TRADE NAME(S):
Betoptic, Betoptic S

THERAPEUTIC CLASS:
Ocular agent

GENERAL USES:
Glaucoma/ocular hypertension

DOSAGE FORMS:
Ophthalmic solution: 0.5%; Ophthalmic suspension: 0.25%

BETAXOLOL (ORAL)
be TAKS oh lol

TRADE NAME(S):
Kerlone

THERAPEUTIC CLASS:
Antihypertensive

GENERAL USES:
Hypertension

DOSAGE FORMS:
Tablets: 10 mg, 20 mg

BEVACIZUMAB
be va SIZ yoo mab
TRADE NAME(S):
Avastin
THERAPEUTIC CLASS:
Antineoplastic
GENERAL USES:
Metastatic colorectal
cancer
DOSAGE FORMS:
Injection: 100 mg, 400 mg

BEXAROTENE
beks AIR oh teen
TRADE NAME(S):
Targretin
THERAPEUTIC CLASS:
Antineoplastic
GENERAL USES:
T-cell lymphoma
DOSAGE FORMS:
Capsules: 75 mg;
Gel: 1%

BICALUTAMIDE
bye ka LOO ta mide
TRADE NAME(S):
Casodex
THERAPEUTIC CLASS:
Antiandrogen
antineoplastic
GENERAL USES:
Prostate cancer
DOSAGE FORMS:
Tablets: 50 mg

BIMATOPROST
bi MAT oh prost
TRADE NAME(S):
Lumigan, Latisse
THERAPEUTIC CLASS:
Ocular agent
GENERAL USES:
Ocular hypertension,
open-angle glaucoma,
promote eyelash growth
DOSAGE FORMS:
Topical and Ophthalmic
solution: 0.03%;
Ophthalmic
solution: 0.01%

BIPERIDEN
bye PER i den
TRADE NAME(S):
Akineton
THERAPEUTIC CLASS:
Antiparkinson agent
GENERAL USES:
Parkinson's disease,
drug-induced
extrapyramidal
disorders
DOSAGE FORMS:
Tablets: 2 mg

BISMUTH SUBCITRATE POTASSIUM/ METRONIDAZOLE/ TETRACYCLINE
BIZ muth/me troe NI da
zole/tet ra SYE kleen
TRADE NAME(S):
Pylera

THERAPEUTIC CLASS:
Anti-infective
GENERAL USES:
Helicobacter pylori
infection-related ulcers
DOSAGE FORMS:
Capsules: 140 mg/
125 mg/125 mg

BISOPROLOL
bis OH proe lol
TRADE NAME(S):
Zebeta
THERAPEUTIC CLASS:
Antihypertensive
GENERAL USES:
Hypertension
DOSAGE FORMS:
Tablets: 5 mg, 10 mg

BISOPROLOL/HCTZ
bis OH proe lol/hye droe klor
oh THYE a zide
TRADE NAME(S):
Ziac
THERAPEUTIC CLASS:
Antihypertensive/
diuretic
GENERAL USES:
Hypertension
DOSAGE FORMS:
Tablets: 2.5 mg/6.25 mg,
5 mg/6.25 mg, 10 mg/
6.25 mg

BITOLTEROL
bye TOLE ter ole
TRADE NAME(S):
Tornalate

THERAPEUTIC CLASS:
Bronchodilator
GENERAL USES:
Bronchospasm/asthma
DOSAGE FORMS:
Inhalation solution: 0.2%;
Aerosol: 0.8%

BIVALIRUDIN
bye VAL i roo din
TRADE NAME(S):
Angiomax
THERAPEUTIC CLASS:
Anticoagulant
GENERAL USES:
Prevent clotting in
angina/PTCA
DOSAGE FORMS:
Injection: 250 mg

BOCEPREVIR
boe SE pre veer
TRADE NAME(S):
Victrelis
THERAPEUTIC CLASS:
Antiviral
GENERAL USES:
Chronic hepatitis C
DOSAGE FORMS:
Capsules: 200 mg

BORTEZOMIB
bore TEZ oh mib
TRADE NAME(S):
Velcade
THERAPEUTIC CLASS:
Antineoplastic

GENERAL USES:
   Multiple myeloma
DOSAGE FORMS:
   Injection: 3.5 mg

BOSENTAN
boe SEN tan
TRADE NAME(S):
   Tracleer
THERAPEUTIC CLASS:
   Cardiac agent
GENERAL USES:
   Pulmonary hypertension
DOSAGE FORMS:
   Tablets: 62.5 mg, 125 mg

BOSUTINIB
boss YOO ti nib
TRADE NAME(S):
   Bosulif
THERAPEUTIC CLASS:
   Antineoplastic
GENERAL USES:
   CML
DOSAGE FORMS:
   Tablets: 100 mg, 500 mg

BRENTUXIMAB VEDOTIN
bren TUX i mab ve DOE tin
TRADE NAME(S):
   Adcetris
THERAPEUTIC CLASS:
   Antineoplastic
GENERAL USES:
   Hodgkin's lymphoma
DOSAGE FORMS:
   Injection: 50 mg

BRIMONIDINE (OPHTHALMIC)
bri MO ni deen
TRADE NAME(S):
   Alphagan, Alphagan P
THERAPEUTIC CLASS:
   Ocular agent
GENERAL USES:
   Glaucoma/ocular hypertension
DOSAGE FORMS:
   Ophthalmic solution: 0.1%, 0.15%, 0.2%

BRIMONIDINE TARTRATE (TOPICAL)
bri MO ni deen
TRADE NAME(S):
   Mirvaso
THERAPEUTIC CLASS:
   Alpha agonist
GENERAL USES:
   Rosacea
DOSAGE FORMS:
   Gel: 0.33%

BRIMONIDINE TARTRATE/ BRINZOLAMIDE
bri MO ni deen/brin ZOE la mide
TRADE NAME(S):
   Simbrinza
THERAPEUTIC CLASS:
   Ocular agent
GENERAL USES:
   Glaucoma, ocular hypertension

DOSAGE FORMS:
Ophthalmic suspension:
0.1%/0.2%

**BRIMONIDINE/
TIMOLOL**
bri MO ni seen/TYE
moe lole
TRADE NAME(S):
Combigan
THERAPEUTIC CLASS:
Ocular agent
GENERAL USES:
Glaucoma, ocular
hypertension
DOSAGE FORMS:
Ophthalmic solution:
0.2%/0.5%

BRINZOLAMIDE
brin ZOH la mide
TRADE NAME(S):
Azopt
THERAPEUTIC CLASS:
Ocular agent
GENERAL USES:
Glaucoma/ocular
hypertension
DOSAGE FORMS:
Ophthalmic solution:
1%

BROMFENAC
BROME fen ak
TRADE NAME(S):
Bromday, Prolensa
THERAPEUTIC CLASS:
Ocular agent

GENERAL USES:
Postoperative cataract
surgery
DOSAGE FORMS:
Ophthalmic solution:
0.07%, 0.09%

BROMOCRIPTINE
broe moe KRIP teen
TRADE NAME(S):
Cycloset, Parlodel
THERAPEUTIC CLASS:
Antiparkinson
agent, antidiabetic
GENERAL USES:
Parkinson's
disease, diabetes (type 2)
DOSAGE FORMS:
Tablets: 0.8 mg, 2.5 mg;
Capsules: 5 mg

BUDESONIDE
byoo DES oh nide
TRADE NAME(S):
Entocort EC, Ucoris
THERAPEUTIC CLASS:
Corticosteroid
GENERAL USES:
Crohn's disease,
ulcerative colitis
DOSAGE FORMS:
Capsules: 3 mg; Extended-
release tablets: 9 mg

BUDESONIDE (INHALED)
byoo DES oh nide
TRADE NAME(S):
Pulmicort

THERAPEUTIC CLASS:
Corticosteroid (inhaler)
GENERAL USES:
Asthma (chronic)
DOSAGE FORMS:
Inhaler: 200 mcg/
inhalation; Inhalation
suspension: 0.25 mg/
2 mL, 0.5 mg/2 mL

BUDESONIDE (NASAL)
byoo DES oh nide
TRADE NAME(S):
Rhinocort, Rhinocort Aqua
THERAPEUTIC CLASS:
Corticosteroid (nasal)
GENERAL USES:
Allergies
DOSAGE FORMS:
Nasal aerosol: 32 mcg/
spray

BUDESONIDE/ FORMOTEROL
byoo DES oh nide/for MOE
te rol
TRADE NAME(S):
Symbicort
THERAPEUTIC CLASS:
Corticosteroid/
bronchodilator
GENERAL USES:
Asthma, COPD
DOSAGE FORMS:
Oral inhalation: 80 mcg/
4.5 mcg/inhalation,
160 mcg/4.5 mcg/
inhalation

BUMETANIDE
byoo MET a nide
TRADE NAME(S):
Bumex
THERAPEUTIC CLASS:
Diuretic
GENERAL USES:
CHF-related edema,
hypertension
DOSAGE FORMS:
Tablets: 0.5 mg, 1 mg,
2 mg; Injection: 0.5 mg,
1 mg, 2.5 mg

BUPIVACAINE (LIPOSOME)
byoo PIV a kane
TRADE NAME(S):
Exparel
THERAPEUTIC CLASS:
Anesthetic
GENERAL USES:
Anesthesia
DOSAGE FORMS:
Injection: 133 mg, 266 mg

BUPRENORPHINE (SUBLINGUAL)
byoo pre NOR feen
TRADE NAME(S):
Subutex, Buprenex
THERAPEUTIC CLASS:
Analgesic (narcotic)
GENERAL USES:
Opioid dependence
DOSAGE FORMS:
Tablets, sublingual: 2 mg,
8 mg; Injection: 0.3 mg

BUPRENORPHINE (TRANSDERMAL)
byoo pre NOR feen

Trade Name(s):
Butrans

Therapeutic Class:
Analgesic

General Uses:
Pain

Dosage Forms:
Patch: 5 mcg/hr, 10 mcg/hr, 20 mcg/hr

BUPRENORPHINE/ NALOXONE (BUCCAL)
byoo pre NOR feen/nal OKS one

Trade Name(s):
Bunavail

Therapeutic Class:
Analgesic (narcotic)/ antidote

General Uses:
Opioid dependence

Dosage Forms:
Buccal film: 2.1 mg/0.3 mg, 4.2 mg/0.7 mg, 6.3 mg/1 mg

BUPRENORPHINE/ NALOXONE (SUBLINGUAL)
byoo pre NOR feen/nal OKS one

Trade Name(s):
Suboxone, Zubsolv

Therapeutic Class:
Analgesic (narcotic)/ narcotic antagonist

General Uses:
Opioid dependence

Dosage Forms:
Film and Tablets, sublingual: 2 mg/0.5 mg, 8 mg/2 mg; Film, sublingual: 4 mg/1 mg, 12 mg/3 mg; Tablets sublingual: 1.4 mg/0.36 mg, 5.7 mg/1.4 mg

BUPROPION
byoo PROE pee on

Trade Name(s):
Wellbutrin, Wellbutrin SR, Wellbutrin XL, Budeprion SR, Aplenzin

Therapeutic Class:
Antidepressant

General Uses:
Depression, seasonal affective disorder

Dosage Forms:
Tablets: 75 mg, 100 mg; Sustained-release tablets: 100 mg, 150 mg, 200 mg; Extended-release tablets: 150 mg, 174 mg, 300 mg, 348 mg, 522 mg

BUPROPION
byoo PROE pee on

Trade Name(s):
Zyban, Buproban

THERAPEUTIC CLASS:
Smoking deterrent
GENERAL USES:
Smoking cessation
DOSAGE FORMS:
Sustained-release tablets:
150 mg

**BUPROPION/
NALTREXONE**
byoo PROE pee on/nal
TREX one
TRADE NAME(S):
Contrave
THERAPEUTIC CLASS:
Anti-obesity agent
GENERAL USES:
Obesity
DOSAGE FORMS:
Extended-release tablets:
90 mg/8 mg

BUSPIRONE
byoo SPYE rone
TRADE NAME(S):
BuSpar
THERAPEUTIC CLASS:
Antianxiety agent
GENERAL USES:
Depression
DOSAGE FORMS:
Tablets: 5 mg, 10 mg,
15 mg, 30 mg

BUTABARBITAL
byoo ta BAR bi tal
TRADE NAME(S):
Butisol

THERAPEUTIC CLASS:
Sedative/hypnotic
GENERAL USES:
Insomnia (short-term
therapy)
DOSAGE FORMS:
Tablets: 15 mg, 30 mg,
50 mg, 100 mg; Elixir:
30 mg/5 mL

BUTENAFINE
byoo TEN a feen
TRADE NAME(S):
Mentax
THERAPEUTIC CLASS:
Antifungal (topical)
GENERAL USES:
Athlete's foot
DOSAGE FORMS:
Cream: 1%

CABAZITAXEL
ka BAZ i TAX el
TRADE NAME(S):
Jevtana
THERAPEUTIC CLASS:
Antineoplastic
GENERAL USES:
Metastatic prostate cancer
DOSAGE FORMS:
Injection: 60 mg

CABERGOLINE
ca BER goe leen
TRADE NAME(S):
Dostinex
THERAPEUTIC CLASS:
Dopamine receptor
agonist

General Uses:
   Hyperprolactinemia
Dosage Forms:
   Tablets: 0.5 mg

**CABOZANTINIB
S-MALEATE**
KA boe ZAN ti nib
Trade Name(s):
   Cometriq
Therapeutic Class:
   Antineoplastic
General Uses:
   Thyroid cancer
Dosage Forms:
   Capsules: 20 mg, 80 mg

CALCIPOTRIENE
kal si POE try een
Trade Name(s):
   Dovonex
Therapeutic Class:
   Antipsoriatic (topical)
General Uses:
   Psoriasis
Dosage Forms:
   Ointment, Solution, and
   Cream: 0.005%

**CALCIPOTRIENE/
BETAMETHASONE
DIPROPIONATE**
kal si POE try een/bay ta
METH a sone
Trade Name(s):
   Taclonex

Therapeutic Class:
   Dermatological agent
General Uses:
   Psoriasis
Dosage Forms:
   Ointment and
   Topical suspension:
   0.005%/0.064%

CALCITONIN
kal si TOE nin
Trade Name(s):
   Miacalcin
Therapeutic Class:
   Hormone
General Uses:
   Osteoporosis, Paget's
   disease
Dosage Forms:
   Injection:
   400 international
   units (IU); Nasal spray:
   200 IU/actuation

**CALCITONIN-SALMON
(rDNA ORIGIN)**
kal si TOE nin
Trade Name(s):
   Fortical
Therapeutic Class:
   Hormone
General Uses:
   Postmenopausal
   osteoporosis
Dosage Forms:
   Nasal spray:
   200 international units/
   actuation

CALCITRIOL (TOPICAL)
kal si TRYE ole
TRADE NAME(S):
Vectical
THERAPEUTIC CLASS:
Vitamin D analog
GENERAL USES:
Plaque psoriasis
DOSAGE FORMS:
Ointment: 3 mcg

CALCIUM CHLORIDE
KAL see um KLOR ide
TRADE NAME(S):
Calcium Chloride
THERAPEUTIC CLASS:
Electrolyte
GENERAL USES:
Replacement
DOSAGE FORMS:
Injection: 10%

CALCIUM GLUCONATE
KAL see um GLOO koe nate
TRADE NAME(S):
Calcium Gluconate
THERAPEUTIC CLASS:
Electrolyte
GENERAL USES:
Replacement
DOSAGE FORMS:
Injection: 10%

CANAGLIFLOZIN
KAN a gli FLOE zin
TRADE NAME(S):
Invokana
THERAPEUTIC CLASS:
Antidiabetic agent

GENERAL USES:
Diabetes (type 2)
DOSAGE FORMS:
Tablets: 100 mg, 300 mg

CANAGLIFLOZIN/ METFORMIN
KAN a gli FLOE zin/MET for min
TRADE NAME(S):
Invokamet
THERAPEUTIC CLASS:
Antidiabetic
GENERAL USES:
Diabetes (type 2)
DOSAGE FORMS:
Tablets: 50 mg/500 mg, 50 mg/1000 mg, 150 mg/500 mg, 150 mg/1000 mg

CANAKINUMAB
KAN a KIN yoo mab
TRADE NAME(S):
Ilaris
THERAPEUTIC CLASS:
Interleukin blocker
GENERAL USES:
Sytemic juvenile idiopathic arthritis, cryopyrin-associated periodic syndromes
DOSAGE FORMS:
Injection: 180 mg

CANDESARTAN
kan de SAR tan
TRADE NAME(S):
Atacand

Therapeutic Class:
Antihypertensive
General Uses:
Hypertension, CHF
Dosage Forms:
Tablets: 4 mg, 8 mg,
16 mg, 32 mg

CAPECITABINE
ka pe SITE a been
Trade Name(s):
Xeloda
Therapeutic Class:
Antineoplastic
General Uses:
Metastatic breast
cancer
Dosage Forms:
Tablets: 150 mg,
500 mg

CAPSAICIN (TRANSDERMAL)
kap SAY sin
Trade Name(s):
Qutenza
Therapeutic Class:
Analgesic
General Uses:
Postherpetic neuralgia
Dosage Forms:
Patch: 8%

CAPTOPRIL
KAP toe pril
Trade Name(s):
Capoten

Therapeutic Class:
Antihypertensive,
cardiac agent
General Uses:
Hypertension, heart
failure, left ventricular
dysfunction, diabetic renal
dysfunction
Dosage Forms:
Tablets: 12.5 mg, 25 mg,
50 mg, 100 mg

CAPTOPRIL/HCTZ
KAP toe pril/hye droe klor oh
THYE a zide
Trade Name(s):
Capozide
Therapeutic Class:
Antihypertensive/
diuretic
General Uses:
Hypertension
Dosage Forms:
Tablets: 25 mg/15 mg,
50 mg/15 mg, 25 mg/
25 mg, 50 mg/25 mg

CARBAMAZEPINE
kar ba MAZ e peen
Trade Name(s):
Tegretol, Epitol,
Equetro
Therapeutic Class:
Anticonvulsant
General Uses:
Seizures, trigeminal
neuralgia

DOSAGE FORMS:
Chewable tablets:
100 mg; Tablets: 200 mg;
Extended-release
tablets: 100 mg, 200 mg,
400 mg; Extended-release
capsules: 100 mg,
200 mg, 300 mg;
Suspension: 100 mg/5 mL

CARBENICILLIN
kar ben i SIL in
TRADE NAME(S):
Geocillin
THERAPEUTIC CLASS:
Anti-infective
GENERAL USES:
Bacterial infections
DOSAGE FORMS:
Tablets: 382 mg

CARBIDOPA/LEVODOPA/ENTACAPONE
kar bi DOE pa/lee voe DOE
pa/en TA ka pone
TRADE NAME(S):
Stalevo
THERAPEUTIC CLASS:
Antiparkinson agent
GENERAL USES:
Parkinson's disease
DOSAGE FORMS:
Tablets: 12.5 mg/
50 mg/200 mg, 25 mg/
100 mg/200 mg, 37.5 mg/
150 mg/200 mg

CARBINOXAMINE MALEATE
kar bi NOKS a meen
TRADE NAME(S):
Karbinal ER
THERAPEUTIC CLASS:
Antihistamine
GENERAL USES:
Allergic reactions,
allergies
DOSAGE FORMS:
Extended-release oral
suspension: 4 mg/5 mL;
Tablets: 4 mg

CARFILZOMIB
car FIL zoe mib
TRADE NAME(S):
Kyprolis
THERAPEUTIC CLASS:
Antineoplastic
GENERAL USES:
Multiple myeloma
DOSAGE FORMS:
Injection: 60 mg

CARGLUMIC ACID
kar GLOO mik AS id
TRADE NAME(S):
Carbaglu
THERAPEUTIC CLASS:
Carbamoyl phosphate
synthetase 1 (CPS 1)
activator
GENERAL USES:
Hyperammonemia
DOSAGE FORMS:
Tablets: 200 mg

CARISOPRODOL
kar i soe PROE dole

TRADE NAME(S):
Soma

THERAPEUTIC CLASS:
Skeletal muscle relaxant

GENERAL USES:
Musculoskeletal
conditions

DOSAGE FORMS:
Tablets: 250 mg, 350 mg

CARTEOLOL (OCULAR)
KAR tee oh lole

TRADE NAME(S):
Ocupress

THERAPEUTIC CLASS:
Ocular agent

GENERAL USES:
Glaucoma/ocular
hypertension

DOSAGE FORMS:
Ophthalmic solution: 1%

CARTEOLOL (ORAL)
KAR tee oh lole

TRADE NAME(S):
Cartrol

THERAPEUTIC CLASS:
Antihypertensive

GENERAL USES:
Hypertension

DOSAGE FORMS:
Tablets: 2.5 mg, 5 mg

CARVEDILOL
KAR ve dil ole

TRADE NAME(S):
Coreg, Coreg CR

THERAPEUTIC CLASS:
Antihypertensive,
cardiac agent

GENERAL USES:
Hypertension, CHF

DOSAGE FORMS:
Tablets: 3.125 mg,
6.25 mg, 12.5 mg, 25 mg;
Extended-release
capsules:
10 mg, 20 mg, 40 mg,
80 mg

CASPOFUNGIN ACETATE
kas poe FUN jin

TRADE NAME(S):
Cancidas

THERAPEUTIC CLASS:
Antifungal

GENERAL USES:
Refractory aspergillosis
infection

DOSAGE FORMS:
Injection: 50 mg, 70 mg

CEFACLOR
SEF a klor

TRADE NAME(S):
Ceclor

THERAPEUTIC CLASS:
Anti-infective

GENERAL USES:
Bacterial infections

Dosage Forms:
Capsules: 250 mg,
500 mg; Extended-release
tablets: 375 mg, 500 mg;
Suspension: 125 mg/
5 mL, 187 mg/5 mL,
250 mg/5 mL, 375 mg/
5 mL; Chewable tablets:
125 mg, 187 mg, 250 mg,
350 mg

CEFADROXIL
sef a DROKS il
Trade Name(s):
Duricef
Therapeutic Class:
Anti-infective
General Uses:
Bacterial infections
Dosage Forms:
Capsules: 500 mg;
Tablets: 1 g; Suspension:
125 mg/5 mL,
250 mg/5 mL,
500 mg/5 mL

CEFAMANDOLE
sef a MAN dole
Trade Name(s):
Mandol
Therapeutic Class:
Anti-infective
General Uses:
Bacterial infections
Dosage Forms:
Injection: 1 g, 2 g

CEFAZOLIN
sef A zoe lin
Trade Name(s):
Ancef, Kefzol
Therapeutic Class:
Anti-infective
General Uses:
Bacterial infections
Dosage Forms:
Injection: 250 mg,
500 mg, 1 g, 5 g, 10 g,
20 g

CEFDINIR
SEF di ner
Trade Name(s):
Omnicef
Therapeutic Class:
Anti-infective
General Uses:
Bacterial infections
Dosage Forms:
Capsules: 300 mg;
Suspension: 125 mg/
5 mL

CEFDITOREN PIVOXIL
sef di TOR en pye VOKS il
Trade Name(s):
Spectracef
Therapeutic Class:
Anti-infective
General Uses:
Bacterial infections
Dosage Forms:
Tablets: 200 mg

CEFEPIME
SEF e pim
TRADE NAME(S):
Maxipime
THERAPEUTIC CLASS:
Anti-infective
GENERAL USES:
Bacterial infections
DOSAGE FORMS:
Injection: 500 mg, 1 g, 2 g

CEFIXIME
sef IKS eem
TRADE NAME(S):
Suprax
THERAPEUTIC CLASS:
Anti-infective
GENERAL USES:
Bacterial infections
DOSAGE FORMS:
Capsules: 400 mg;
Chewable tablets: 100 mg,
150 mg, 200 mg;
Tablets: 400 mg;
Suspension: 100 mg/
5 mL, 200 mg/5 mL,
500 mg/15 mL

CEFMETAZOLE
sef MET ah zole
TRADE NAME(S):
Zefazone
THERAPEUTIC CLASS:
Anti-infective
GENERAL USES:
Bacterial infections
DOSAGE FORMS:
Injection: 1 g, 2 g

CEFONICID
se FON i sid
TRADE NAME(S):
Monocid
THERAPEUTIC CLASS:
Anti-infective
GENERAL USES:
Bacterial infections
DOSAGE FORMS:
Injection: 1 g, 10 g

CEFOPERAZONE
sef oh PER a zone
TRADE NAME(S):
Cefobid
THERAPEUTIC CLASS:
Anti-infective
GENERAL USES:
Bacterial infections
DOSAGE FORMS:
Injection: 1 g, 2 g, 10 g

CEFOTAXIME SODIUM
sef oh TAKS eem
TRADE NAME(S):
Claforan
THERAPEUTIC CLASS:
Anti-infective
GENERAL USES:
Bacterial infections
DOSAGE FORMS:
Injection: 500 mg, 1 g,
2 g, 10 g

CEFOXITIN SODIUM
se FOKS i tin
TRADE NAME(S):
Mefoxin

THERAPEUTIC CLASS:
Anti-infective
GENERAL USES:
Bacterial infections
DOSAGE FORMS:
Injection: 1 g, 2 g, 10 g

CEFPODOXIME
sef pode OKS eem
TRADE NAME(S):
Vantin
THERAPEUTIC CLASS:
Anti-infective
GENERAL USES:
Bacterial infections
DOSAGE FORMS:
Tablets: 100 mg, 200 mg;
Suspension: 50 mg/5 mL,
100 mg/5 mL

CEFPROZIL
sef PROE zil
TRADE NAME(S):
Cefzil
THERAPEUTIC CLASS:
Anti-infective
GENERAL USES:
Bacterial infections
DOSAGE FORMS:
Capsules: 250 mg,
500 mg; Suspension:
125 mg/5 mL, 250 mg/
5 mL

CEFTAROLINE FOSAMIL
sef TAR oh leen FOS a mil
TRADE NAME(S):
Teflaro

THERAPEUTIC CLASS:
Anti-infective
GENERAL USES:
Bacterial infections
DOSAGE FORMS:
Injection: 400 mg, 600 mg

CEFTAZIDIME
SEF tay zi deem
TRADE NAME(S):
Fortaz, Ceptaz, Tazidime
THERAPEUTIC CLASS:
Anti-infective
GENERAL USES:
Bacterial infections
DOSAGE FORMS:
Injection: 500 mg, 1 g,
2 g, 6 g, 10 g

CEFTIBUTEN
sef TYE byoo ten
TRADE NAME(S):
Cedax
THERAPEUTIC CLASS:
Anti-infective
GENERAL USES:
Bacterial infections
DOSAGE FORMS:
Capsules: 400 mg;
Suspension: 90 mg/5 mL,
180 mg/5 mL

CEFTIZOXIME SODIUM
sef ti ZOKS eem
TRADE NAME(S):
Cefizox
THERAPEUTIC CLASS:
Anti-infective

GENERAL USES:
Bacterial infections

DOSAGE FORMS:
Injection: 500 mg, 1 g,
2 g, 10 g

CEFTRIAXONE SODIUM
sef trye AKS one

TRADE NAME(S):
Rocephin

THERAPEUTIC CLASS:
Anti-infective

GENERAL USES:
Bacterial infections

DOSAGE FORMS:
Injection: 250 mg,
500 mg, 1 g, 2 g, 10 g

CEFUROXIME AXETIL
se fyoor OKS eem
AKS e til

TRADE NAME(S):
Ceftin

THERAPEUTIC CLASS:
Anti-infective

GENERAL USES:
Bacterial infections

DOSAGE FORMS:
Tablets: 125 mg, 250 mg,
500 mg; Suspension:
125 mg/5 mL, 250 mg/
5 mL

CEFUROXIME SODIUM
se fyoor OKS eem

TRADE NAME(S):
Zinacef

THERAPEUTIC CLASS:
Anti-infective

GENERAL USES:
Bacterial infections

DOSAGE FORMS:
Injection: 750 mg, 1.5 mg,
7.5 g

CELECOXIB
se le KOKS ib

TRADE NAME(S):
Celebrex

THERAPEUTIC CLASS:
Anti-inflammatory/
analgesic

GENERAL USES:
Osteoarthritis, rheumatoid
arthritis, dysmenorrhea,
FAP, acute pain

DOSAGE FORMS:
Capsules: 100 mg, 200 mg

CEPHALEXIN
sef a LEKS in

TRADE NAME(S):
Keflex, Biocef

THERAPEUTIC CLASS:
Anti-infective

GENERAL USES:
Bacterial infections

DOSAGE FORMS:
Capsules: 250 mg,
333 mg, 500 mg, 750 mg;
Tablets: 250 mg, 500 mg;
Suspension: 125 mg/
5 mL, 250 mg/5 mL

CEPHALEXIN HCL
sef a LEKS in
TRADE NAME(S):
Keftab
THERAPEUTIC CLASS:
Anti-infective
GENERAL USES:
Bacterial infections
DOSAGE FORMS:
Tablets: 500 mg

CEPHRADINE
SEF ra deen
TRADE NAME(S):
Velosef
THERAPEUTIC CLASS:
Anti-infective
GENERAL USES:
Bacterial infections
DOSAGE FORMS:
Capsules: 250 mg,
500 mg; Suspension:
125 mg/5 mL, 250 mg/
5 mL; Injection: 250 mg,
500 mg, 1 g, 2 g

CERITINIB
se RI ti nib
TRADE NAME(S):
Zykadia
THERAPEUTIC CLASS:
Antineoplastic
GENERAL USES:
Lung cancer
DOSAGE FORMS:
Capsules: 150 mg

CERTOLIZUMAB PEGOL
SER toe LIZ oo mab peg OL
TRADE NAME(S):
Cimzia
THERAPEUTIC CLASS:
Tumor necrosis factor,
rheumatoid arthritis,
psoriatic arthritis,
ankylosing spondylitis
GENERAL USES:
Crohn's disease
DOSAGE FORMS:
Injection: 200 mg

CETIRIZINE
se TI ra zeen
TRADE NAME(S):
Zyrtec
THERAPEUTIC CLASS:
Antihistamine
GENERAL USES:
Allergic rhinitis/hives
DOSAGE FORMS:
Tablets and Chewable
tablets: 5 mg, 10 mg;
Orally disintegrating
tablets: 10 mg;
Syrup: 5 mg/5 mL

**CETIRIZINE/
PSEUDOEPHEDRINE**
se TI ra zeen/soo doe e FED
rin
TRADE NAME(S):
Zyrtec-D
THERAPEUTIC CLASS:
Antihistamine/
decongestant

GENERAL USES:
Allergies
DOSAGE FORMS:
Extended-release tablets:
5 mg/120 mg

CETRORELIX ACETATE
set roe REL iks
TRADE NAME(S):
Cetrotide
THERAPEUTIC CLASS:
Hormone antagonist
GENERAL USES:
Prevention of LH surges
DOSAGE FORMS:
Injection: 0.25 mg, 3 mg

CETUXIMAB
se TUK see mab
TRADE NAME(S):
Erbitux
THERAPEUTIC CLASS:
Antineoplastic
GENERAL USES:
Various cancers
DOSAGE FORMS:
Injection: 100 mg

CEVIMELINE
se vi ME leen
TRADE NAME(S):
Evoxac
THERAPEUTIC CLASS:
Saliva stimulant
GENERAL USES:
Dry mouth in Sjögren's
syndrome

DOSAGE FORMS:
Capsules: 30 mg

CHLORAL HYDRATE
KLOR al HYE drate
TRADE NAME(S):
Somnote
THERAPEUTIC CLASS:
Sedative/hypnotic
GENERAL USES:
Pre-op sedation
DOSAGE FORMS:
Capsules: 500 mg

**CHLORAMPHENICOL
(OCULAR)**
klor am FEN i kole
TRADE NAME(S):
AK-Chlor, Chloroptic,
Ocuchlor
THERAPEUTIC CLASS:
Ocular agent
(anti-infective)
GENERAL USES:
Ocular infections
DOSAGE FORMS:
Ophthalmic solution:
5 mg/mL; Ophthalmic
ointment: 10 mg/g

**CHLORAMPHENICOL
(ORAL)**
klor am FEN i kole
TRADE NAME(S):
Chloromycetin
THERAPEUTIC CLASS:
Anti-infective

GENERAL USES:
Bacterial infections
DOSAGE FORMS:
Capsules: 250 mg;
Injection: 1 g

CHLORDIAZEPOXIDE
klor dye az e POKS ide
TRADE NAME(S):
Librium, Mitran, Libritabs
THERAPEUTIC CLASS:
Antianxiety agent,
anticonvulsant
GENERAL USES:
Anxiety, alcohol
withdrawal, seizures
DOSAGE FORMS:
Capsules: 5 mg, 10 mg,
25 mg; Tablets: 10 mg,
25 mg; Injection: 100 mg

CHLORDIAZEPOXIDE/ AMITRIPTYLINE
klor dye az e POKS ide/a
mee TRIP ti leen
TRADE NAME(S):
Limbitrol DS
THERAPEUTIC CLASS:
Sedative/antidepressant
GENERAL USES:
Depression/anxiety
DOSAGE FORMS:
Tablets: 5 mg/12.5 mg,
10 mg/25 mg

CHLOROQUINE PHOSPHATE
KLOR oh kwin
TRADE NAME(S):
Aralen
THERAPEUTIC CLASS:
Antimalarial
GENERAL USES:
Malaria treatment
and prevention,
intestinal
amebiasis
DOSAGE FORMS:
Tablets: 250 mg, 500 mg

CHLOROTHIAZIDE
klor oh THYE a zide
TRADE NAME(S):
Diuril
THERAPEUTIC CLASS:
Diuretic
GENERAL USES:
CHF-related edema,
hypertension
DOSAGE FORMS:
Tablets: 250 mg, 500 mg;
Suspension: 250 mg/
5 mL

CHLORPROMAZINE
klor PROE ma zeen
TRADE NAME(S):
Thorazine
THERAPEUTIC CLASS:
Antipsychotic
GENERAL USES:
Psychotic/behavioral

disorders, porphyria, emesis

DOSAGE FORMS:
Tablets: 10 mg, 25 mg, 50 mg, 100 mg, 200 mg; Sustained-release capsules: 30 mg, 75 mg, 150 mg, 200 mg, 300 mg; Syrup: 10 mg/5 mL; Concentrated solution: 30 mg/mL, 100 mg/mL; Injection: 25 mg, 50 mg

CHLORPROPAMIDE
klor PROE pa mide
TRADE NAME(S):
Diabinese
THERAPEUTIC CLASS:
Antidiabetic
GENERAL USES:
Diabetes (type 2)
DOSAGE FORMS:
Tablets: 100 mg, 250 mg

CHLORTHALIDONE
klor THAL i done
TRADE NAME(S):
Thalitone, Hygroton
THERAPEUTIC CLASS:
Diuretic
GENERAL USES:
CHF-related edema, hypertension
DOSAGE FORMS:
Tablets: 15 mg, 25 mg, 50 mg, 100 mg

CHLORZOXAZONE
klor ZOKS a zone
TRADE NAME(S):
Paraflex, Parafon Forte DSC, Remular
THERAPEUTIC CLASS:
Skeletal muscle relaxant
GENERAL USES:
Musculoskeletal conditions
DOSAGE FORMS:
Tablets and Capsules: 250 mg, 500 mg

CHOLINE C 11
KOE leen
TRADE NAME(S):
Choline C 11
THERAPEUTIC CLASS:
Diagnostic agent
GENERAL USES:
PET imaging for prostate cancer
DOSAGE FORMS:
Injection: 148 to 1225 MBq/mL

CHOLINE FENOFIBRATE
KOE leen FEN oh FYE brate
TRADE NAME(S):
Trilipix
THERAPEUTIC CLASS:
Antilipemic
GENERAL USES:
Hyperlipidemia
DOSAGE FORMS:
Delayed-release capsules: 45 mg, 135 mg

CICLESONIDE
sye KLE soh nide
TRADE NAME(S):
  Omnaris, Zetonna
THERAPEUTIC CLASS:
  Corticosteroid
GENERAL USES:
  Seasonal and perennial
  allergies
DOSAGE FORMS:
  Nasal aerosol: 37 mcg;
  Nasal spray: 50 mcg

CICLOPIROX
sye kloe PEER oks
TRADE NAME(S):
  Loprox, Penlac
THERAPEUTIC CLASS:
  Antifungal (topical)
GENERAL USES:
  Athlete's foot, jock itch,
  ringworm, nail infections
  (topical nail preparation)
DOSAGE FORMS:
  Cream and Lotion: 1%;
  Nail lacquer: 8%

CILOSTAZOL
sil OH sta zol
TRADE NAME(S):
  Pletal
THERAPEUTIC CLASS:
  Antiplatelet agent
GENERAL USES:
  Intermittent
  claudication
DOSAGE FORMS:
  Tablets: 50 mg, 100 mg

CIMETIDINE
sye MET i deen
TRADE NAME(S):
  Tagamet, Tagamet HB
THERAPEUTIC CLASS:
  Gastric acid secretion
  inhibitor
GENERAL USES:
  Duodenal ulcer, GERD,
  heartburn (OTC)
DOSAGE FORMS:
  Tablets: 100 mg, 200 mg,
  300 mg, 400 mg, 800 mg;
  Solution: 300 mg/5 mL;
  Injection: 300 mg, 600 mg

CINACALCET
sin a KAL set
TRADE NAME(S):
  Sensipar
THERAPEUTIC CLASS:
  Hyperparathyroid agent
GENERAL USES:
  Secondary
  hyperparathyroidism,
  hypercalcemia in
  parathyroid cancer
DOSAGE FORMS:
  Tablets: 30 mg, 60 mg,
  90 mg

CINOXACIN
sin OKS a sin
TRADE NAME(S):
  Cinobac
THERAPEUTIC CLASS:
  Anti-infective
GENERAL USES:

Bacterial infections

DOSAGE FORMS:
Capsules: 250 mg,
500 mg

CIPROFLOXACIN
sip roe FLOKS a sin
TRADE NAME(S):
Cipro, Cipro XR, Proquin
XR
THERAPEUTIC CLASS:
Anti-infective
GENERAL USES:
Bacterial infections
DOSAGE FORMS:
Tablets: 100 mg, 250 mg,
500 mg, 750 mg;
Extended-release tablets:
500 mg, 1000 mg;
Suspension: 250 mg/
5 mL, 500 mg/5 mL;
Injection: 200 mg, 400 mg

CIPROFLOXACIN (OCULAR)
sip roe FLOKS a sin
TRADE NAME(S):
Ciloxan
THERAPEUTIC CLASS:
Ocular agent
(anti-infective)
GENERAL USES:
Ocular
infections
DOSAGE FORMS:
Ophthalmic solution and
Ointment: 0.3%

CIPROFLOXACIN (OTIC)
sip roe FLOKS a sin
TRADE NAME(S):
Cetraxal
THERAPEUTIC CLASS:
Otic agent (anti-infective)
GENERAL USES:
Ear infections
DOSAGE FORMS:
Otic solution: 0.2%
(0.5 mg/0.25 mL)

CIPROFLOXACIN/ DEXAMETHASONE (OTIC)
sip roe FLOKS a sin/deks a
METH a sone
TRADE NAME(S):
Ciprodex
THERAPEUTIC CLASS:
Otic agent
(anti-infective/
anti-inflammatory)
GENERAL USES:
Acute otitis media
DOSAGE FORMS:
Otic suspension:
0.3%/0.1%

CIPROFLOXACIN/ HYDROCORTISONE (OTIC)
sip roe FLOKS a sin/
hye droe KOR ti sone
TRADE NAME(S):
Cipro HC
THERAPEUTIC CLASS:
Otic agent

(anti-infective/
anti-inflammatory)
GENERAL USES:
Acute otitis media
DOSAGE FORMS:
Otic suspension: 2 mg/
10 mg per mL

CISPLATIN
SIS pla tin
TRADE NAME(S):
Platinol-AQ
THERAPEUTIC CLASS:
Antineoplastic
GENERAL USES:
Cancer of the
bladder, testes,
ovaries
DOSAGE FORMS:
Injection: 50 mg,
100 mg, 200 mg

CITALOPRAM
sye TAL oh pram
TRADE NAME(S):
Celexa
THERAPEUTIC CLASS:
Antidepressant
GENERAL USES:
Depression, anxiety
DOSAGE FORMS:
Tablets: 10 mg, 20 mg,
40 mg; Solution: 10 mg/
5 mL

CLARITHROMYCIN
kla RITH roe mye sin
TRADE NAME(S):
Biaxin, Biaxin XL

THERAPEUTIC CLASS:
Anti-infective
GENERAL USES:
Bacterial
infections
DOSAGE FORMS:
Tablets: 250 mg; Tablets
and Extended-release
tablets: 500 mg;
Suspension: 125 mg/
5 mL, 250 mg/5 mL

CLEVIDIPINE BUTYRATE
kle VID i peen
TRADE NAME(S):
Cleviprex
THERAPEUTIC CLASS:
Antihypertensive
GENERAL USES:
Hypertension
DOSAGE FORMS:
Injection: 25 mg, 50 mg

CLINDAMYCIN
klin da MYE sin
TRADE NAME(S):
Cleocin
THERAPEUTIC CLASS:
Anti-infective
GENERAL USES:
Bacterial infections
DOSAGE FORMS:
Capsules: 75 mg, 150 mg,
300 mg; Solution: 75 mg/
5 mL; Injection: 300 mg,
600 mg, 900 mg

CLINDAMYCIN (TOPICAL)
klin da MYE sin

TRADE NAME(S):
Cleocin T, Clinda-Derm

THERAPEUTIC CLASS:
Anti-infective (topical)

GENERAL USES:
Acne

DOSAGE FORMS:
Gel, Lotion, and Topical
solution: 10 mg/mL

CLINDAMYCIN (VAGINAL)
klin da MYE sin

TRADE NAME(S):
Cleocin, Clindesse

THERAPEUTIC CLASS:
Vaginal anti-infective

GENERAL USES:
Vaginal bacterial
infections

DOSAGE FORMS:
Cream: 2%

CLINDAMYCIN/ TRETINOIN (TOPICAL)
klin da MYE sin/ TRET i
noyn

TRADE NAME(S):
Veltin

THERAPEUTIC CLASS:
Anti-infective/retinoid

GENERAL USES:
Acne

DOSAGE FORMS:
Gel: 1.2%/0.025%

CLOBAZAM
KLOE ba zam

TRADE NAME(S):
Onfi

THERAPEUTIC CLASS:
Anticonvulsant

GENERAL USES:
Seizures

DOSAGE FORMS:
Tablets: 10 mg, 20 mg;
Suspension: 2.5 mg/mL

CLOBETASOL
kloe BAY ta sol

TRADE NAME(S):
Temovate, Olux-E

THERAPEUTIC CLASS:
Corticosteroid (topical)

GENERAL USES:
Various skin conditions

DOSAGE FORMS:
Ointment, Cream, Foam,
Gel, Lotion, Solution,
Shampoo, and Topical
spray: 0.05%

CLOFARABINE
kloe FAR a been

TRADE NAME(S):
Clolar

THERAPEUTIC CLASS:
Antineoplastic

GENERAL USES:
Pediatric cancer (ALL)

DOSAGE FORMS:
Injection: 20 mg

CLOMIPRAMINE
kloe MI pra meen
TRADE NAME(S):
Anafranil
THERAPEUTIC CLASS:
Antidepressant
GENERAL USES:
OCD
DOSAGE FORMS:
Capsules: 25 mg, 50 mg,
75 mg

CLONAZEPAM
kloe NA ze pam
TRADE NAME(S):
Klonopin
THERAPEUTIC CLASS:
Anticonvulsant
GENERAL USES:
Seizures
DOSAGE FORMS:
Tablets: 0.5 mg, 1 mg,
2 mg

CLONIDINE
KLON i deen
TRADE NAME(S):
Catapres, Catapres-TTS
THERAPEUTIC CLASS:
Antihypertensive
GENERAL USES:
Hypertension
DOSAGE FORMS:
Tablets: 0.1 mg, 0.2 mg,
0.3 mg; Transdermal
patch (content): 2.5 mg,
5 mg, 7.5 mg

CLONIDINE
KLON i deen
TRADE NAME(S):
Kapvay
THERAPEUTIC CLASS:
ADHD agent
GENERAL USES:
ADHD
DOSAGE FORMS:
Extended-release tablets:
0.1 mg, 0.2 mg

**CLONIDINE/
CHLORTHALIDONE**
KLON i deen/klor THAL i
done
TRADE NAME(S):
Combipres
THERAPEUTIC CLASS:
Antihypertensive/diuretic
GENERAL USES:
Hypertension
DOSAGE FORMS:
Tablets: 0.1 mg/15 mg,
0.2 mg/15 mg, 0.3 mg/
15 mg

CLOPIDOGREL
kloh PID oh grel
TRADE NAME(S):
Plavix
THERAPEUTIC CLASS:
Antiplatelet agent
GENERAL USES:
Reduce stroke, MI risk,
acute coronary syndrome
DOSAGE FORMS:
Tablets: 75 mg

CLORAZEPATE
klor AZ e pate

TRADE NAME(S):
Tranxene, Gen-Xene

THERAPEUTIC CLASS:
Antianxiety agent, anticonvulsant

GENERAL USES:
Anxiety, panic disorder, seizures

DOSAGE FORMS:
Capsules or Tablets:
3.75 mg, 7.5 mg, 15 mg;
Single-dose tablets:
11.25 mg, 22.5 mg

CLOTRIMAZOLE (ORAL)
kloe TRIM a zole

TRADE NAME(S):
Mycelex

THERAPEUTIC CLASS:
Antifungal

GENERAL USES:
Oral fungal infection
(candidiasis)

DOSAGE FORMS:
Troches: 10 mg

CLOTRIMAZOLE (TOPICAL)
kloe TRIM a zole

TRADE NAME(S):
Lotrimin, Mycelex

THERAPEUTIC CLASS:
Antifungal (topical)

GENERAL USES:
Athlete's foot, jock itch, ringworm, tinea versicolor, candidiasis

DOSAGE FORMS:
Cream, Solution, and
Lotion: 1%

CLOXACILLIN
kloks a SIL in

TRADE NAME(S):
Cloxapen

THERAPEUTIC CLASS:
Anti-infective

GENERAL USES:
Bacterial infections

DOSAGE FORMS:
Capsules: 250 mg,
500 mg; Solution:
125 mg/5 mL

CLOZAPINE
KLOE za peen

TRADE NAME(S):
Clozaril, Versacloz

THERAPEUTIC CLASS:
Antipsychotic

GENERAL USES:
Psychotic
disorders

DOSAGE FORMS:
Tablets: 25 mg,
100 mg, 200 mg; Orally
disintegrating tablets:
25 mg, 100 mg;
Suspension: 50 mg/mL

COBICISTAT
koe BIK i stat

TRADE NAME(S):
Tybost

THERAPEUTIC CLASS:
Anti-infective agent
GENERAL USES:
HIV infection
DOSAGE FORMS:
Tablets: 150 mg

CODEINE SULFATE
KOE deen
TRADE NAME(S):
Codeine
THERAPEUTIC CLASS:
Analgesic (narcotic)
GENERAL USES:
Pain, cough
DOSAGE FORMS:
Tablets: 15 mg, 30 mg,
60 mg; Soluble tablets:
30 mg, 60 mg

COLCHICINE
KOL chi seen
TRADE NAME(S):
Colcrys, Mitigare
THERAPEUTIC CLASS:
Antineoplastic
GENERAL USES:
Gout, familial
Mediterranean fever
DOSAGE FORMS:
Tablets: 0.6 mg

COLESEVELAM
koh le SEV a lam
TRADE NAME(S):
Welchol
THERAPEUTIC CLASS:
Antilipemic

GENERAL USES:
Hyperlipidemia
DOSAGE FORMS:
Suspension (oral): 1.875 g,
3.75 g; Tablets: 625 mg

COLLAGENASE CLOSTRIDIUM HISTOLYTICUM
COL a geh nase klo STRID
ee um his toe LIT ik um
TRADE NAME(S):
Xiaflex
THERAPEUTIC CLASS:
Miscellaneous
GENERAL USES:
Dupuytren's contracture,
Peyronie's disease
DOSAGE FORMS:
Injection: 0.9 mg

CONIVAPTAN
koe NYE vap tan
TRADE NAME(S):
Vaprisol
THERAPEUTIC CLASS:
Vasopressin receptor
antagonist
GENERAL USES:
Euvolemic hyponatremia
DOSAGE FORMS:
Injection: 20 mg

CRIZOTINIB
kriz OH ti nib
TRADE NAME(S):
Xalkori

THERAPEUTIC CLASS:
Antineoplastic
GENERAL USES:
Non-small-cell lung
cancer
DOSAGE FORMS:
Capsules: 200 mg, 250 mg

CROFELEMER
kroe FEL e mer
TRADE NAME(S):
Fulyzaq
THERAPEUTIC CLASS:
Anti-diarrheal
GENERAL USES:
Diarrhea in HIV/AIDS
patients on anti-retroviral
therapy
DOSAGE FORMS:
Delayed-release tablets:
125 mg

CROMOLYN (INHALED)
KROE moe lin
TRADE NAME(S):
Intal
THERAPEUTIC CLASS:
Respiratory inhalant
GENERAL USES:
Asthma, bronchospasm
DOSAGE FORMS:
Aerosol spray: 800 mcg/
spray; Nebulizer solution:
20 mg/2 mL

CROMOLYN (OCULAR)
KROE moe lin
TRADE NAME(S):
Crolom
THERAPEUTIC CLASS:
Ocular agent
GENERAL USES:
Conjunctivitis
DOSAGE FORMS:
Ophthalmic solution: 4%

CROMOLYN (ORAL)
KROE moe lin
TRADE NAME(S):
Gastrocrom
THERAPEUTIC CLASS:
Mast cell stabilizer
GENERAL USES:
Mastocytosis
DOSAGE FORMS:
Oral concentrate: 100 mg/
5 mL

CROTAMITON
kroe TAM i ton
TRADE NAME(S):
Eurax
THERAPEUTIC CLASS:
Scabicide (topical)
GENERAL USES:
Scabies, pruritus
DOSAGE FORMS:
Cream and Lotion: 10%

CYANOCOBALAMIN
sye an oh koe BAL a min
TRADE NAME(S):
Nascobal, Vitamin B-12

THERAPEUTIC CLASS:
Vitamin
GENERAL USES:
Vitamin B12 deficiency
DOSAGE FORMS:
Nasal gel: 500 mcg/
0.1 mL; Nasal spray:
500 mcg/0.1 mL;
Injection: 1000 mcg/mL;
Tablets: 50 mcg, 100 mcg,
250 mcg, 500 mcg,
1000 mcg, 5000 mcg;
Extended-release tablets:
1500 mcg; Sublingual
tablets: 2500 mcg;
Lozenges: 100 mcg,
250 mcg, 500 mcg

CYCLOBENZAPRINE
sye kloe BEN za preen
TRADE NAME(S):
Flexeril
THERAPEUTIC CLASS:
Skeletal muscle
relaxant
GENERAL USES:
Musculoskeletal
conditions
DOSAGE FORMS:
Tablets: 5 mg, 7.5 mg,
10 mg

CYCLOPHOSPHAMIDE
sye kloe FOS fa mide
TRADE NAME(S):
Cytoxan
THERAPEUTIC CLASS:
Antineoplastic

GENERAL USES:
Various lymphomas and
leukemias, minimal
change nephrotic
syndrome
DOSAGE FORMS:
Tablets: 25 mg, 50 mg;
Injection: 100 mg,
200 mg, 500 mg, 1 g, 2 g;
Capsules: 25 mg, 50 mg

CYCLOSERINE
sye kloe SER een
TRADE NAME(S):
Seromycin
THERAPEUTIC CLASS:
Antituberculosis
agent
GENERAL USES:
Tuberculosis
DOSAGE FORMS:
Capsules: 250 mg

CYCLOSPORINE
SYE kloe spor een
TRADE NAME(S):
Sandimmune, Neoral,
SangCya
THERAPEUTIC CLASS:
Immunosuppressant
GENERAL USES:
Rheumatoid arthritis,
psoriasis, prevent organ
rejection
DOSAGE FORMS:
Capsules: 25 mg, 50 mg,
100 mg; Solution:

100 mg/mL; Injection:
250 mg

CYCLOSPORINE (OCULAR)
SYE kloe spor een

Trade Name(s):
Restasis

Therapeutic Class:
Ocular agent
(anti-inflammatory)

General Uses:
Increase tear production

Dosage Forms:
Ophthalmic emulsion:
0.05%

CYPROHEPTADINE
si proe HEP ta deen

Trade Name(s):
Periactin

Therapeutic Class:
Antihistamine

General Uses:
Allergies

Dosage Forms:
Tablets: 4 mg; Syrup:
2 mg/5 mL

CYSTEAMINE BITARTRATE
sis TEE a meen

Trade Name(s):
Procysbi

Therapeutic Class:
Renal-urologic agent

General Uses:
Nephropathic cystinosis

Dosage Forms:
Delayed-release capsules:
25 mg, 75 mg

CYSTEAMINE HCL
sis TEE a meen

Trade Name(s):
Cystaran

Therapeutic Class:
Ocular agent

General Uses:
Corneal cysteine crystal
accumulation

Dosage Forms:
Ophthalmic solution:
0.44%

DABIGATRAN ETEXILATE MESYLATE
da bye GAT ran e TEX i late
MES i late

Trade Name(s):
Pradaxa

Therapeutic Class:
Thrombin inhibitor

General Uses:
Reduce risk of stroke,
prevent and treat clots

Dosage Forms:
Capsules: 75 mg, 150 mg

DABRAFENIB
da BRAF e nib

Trade Name(s):
Tafinlar

Therapeutic Class:
Antineoplastic

GENERAL USES:
Melanoma
DOSAGE FORMS:
Capsules: 50 mg, 75 mg

DALBAVANCIN
DAL ba VAN sin
TRADE NAME(S):
Dalvance
THERAPEUTIC CLASS:
Anti-infective
GENERAL USES:
Bacterial infections
DOSAGE FORMS:
Injection: 500 mg

DALFAMPRIDINE
dal FAM pri DEEN
TRADE NAME(S):
Ampyra
THERAPEUTIC CLASS:
Potassium channel
blocker
GENERAL USES:
Multiple sclerosis
DOSAGE FORMS:
Extended-release tablets:
10 mg

DALTEPARIN SODIUM
dal TE pa rin
TRADE NAME(S):
Fragmin
THERAPEUTIC CLASS:
Anticoagulant (LMWH)
GENERAL USES:
Prevention of blood clots

DOSAGE FORMS:
Injection:
2500 international units
(IU), 5000 IU, 95,000 IU

DANAPAROID SODIUM
da NAP a roid
TRADE NAME(S):
Orgaran
THERAPEUTIC CLASS:
Anticoagulant
GENERAL USES:
Prevention of blood clots
DOSAGE FORMS:
Injection: 750 anti-Xa
units

DANTROLENE
DAN troe leen
TRADE NAME(S):
Dantrium, Ryanodex
THERAPEUTIC CLASS:
Skeletal muscle relaxant
GENERAL USES:
Spasticity, hyperthermia
DOSAGE FORMS:
Capsules: 25 mg, 50 mg,
100 mg; Injection: 20 mg,
250 mg

DAPAGLIFLOZIN
DAP a gli FLOE zin
TRADE NAME(S):
Farxiga
THERAPEUTIC CLASS:
Antidiabetic agent
GENERAL USES:
Diabetes (type 2)

DOSAGE FORMS:
Tablets: 5 mg, 10 mg

DAPSONE
DAP sone
TRADE NAME(S):
Aczone
THERAPEUTIC CLASS:
Dermatologic agent
GENERAL USES:
Acne vulgaris
DOSAGE FORMS:
Gel: 5%

DAPTOMYCIN
DAP toe mye sin
TRADE NAME(S):
Cubicin
THERAPEUTIC CLASS:
Anti-infective
GENERAL USES:
Bacterial infections
DOSAGE FORMS:
Injection: 250 mg, 500 mg

DARBEPOETIN ALFA
dar be POE e tin AL fa
TRADE NAME(S):
Aranesp
THERAPEUTIC CLASS:
Hematological agent
GENERAL USES:
Anemia
DOSAGE FORMS:
Injection: 0.025 mg,
0.04 mg, 0.06 mg, 0.1 mg,
0.15 mg, 0.2 mg, 0.3 mg,
0.5 mg

DARIFENACIN HYDROBROMIDE
dar i FEN a sin
TRADE NAME(S):
Enablex
THERAPEUTIC CLASS:
Anticholinergic
GENERAL USES:
Overactive bladder
DOSAGE FORMS:
Extended-release tablets:
7.5 mg, 15 mg

DARUNAVIR
da ROO na veer
TRADE NAME(S):
Prezista
THERAPEUTIC CLASS:
Antiviral
GENERAL USES:
HIV infection
DOSAGE FORMS:
Tablets: 75 mg, 150 mg,
400 mg, 600 mg;
Suspension (oral):
100 mg/mL

DASATINIB
da SA ti nib
TRADE NAME(S):
Sprycel
THERAPEUTIC CLASS:
Antineoplastic
GENERAL USES:
Myelogenous leukemia
DOSAGE FORMS:
Tablets: 20 mg, 50 mg,
70 mg

DECITABINE
de SYE ta been
TRADE NAME(S):
  Dacogen
THERAPEUTIC CLASS:
  Antineoplastic
GENERAL USES:
  Myelodysplastic disease
DOSAGE FORMS:
  Injection: 50 mg

DEFERASIROX
de FER a sir oks
TRADE NAME(S):
  Exjade
THERAPEUTIC CLASS:
  Chelating agent
GENERAL USES:
  Chronic iron overload
  DOSAGE FORMS:
  Tablets: 125 mg, 250 mg,
  500 mg

DEFERIPRONE
de FER i prone
TRADE NAME(S):
  Ferriprox
THERAPEUTIC CLASS:
  Chelating agent
GENERAL USES:
  Chronic iron overload due
  to blood transfusions
DOSAGE FORMS:
  Tablets: 500 mg

DEGARELIX ACETATE
DEG a REL ix
TRADE NAME(S):
  Firmagon
THERAPEUTIC CLASS:
  Antineoplastic
GENERAL USES:
  Prostate cancer
DOSAGE FORMS:
  Injection: 80 mg, 120 mg

DELAVIRDINE
de la VEER deen
TRADE NAME(S):
  Rescriptor
THERAPEUTIC CLASS:
  Antiviral
GENERAL USES:
  HIV infection
DOSAGE FORMS:
  Tablets: 100 mg, 200 mg

DEMECARIUM
dem e KARE ee um
TRADE NAME(S):
  Humorsol
THERAPEUTIC CLASS:
  Ocular agent
GENERAL USES:
  Glaucoma
DOSAGE FORMS:
  Ophthalmic solution:
  0.125%, 0.25%

DEMECLOCYCLINE
dem e kloe SYE kleen
TRADE NAME(S):
  Declomycin

THERAPEUTIC CLASS:
Anti-infective
GENERAL USES:
Bacterial infections
DOSAGE FORMS:
Tablets: 150 mg, 300 mg

DENOSUMAB
den OH soo mab
TRADE NAME(S):
Prolia, Xgeva
THERAPEUTIC CLASS:
Receptor activator for
nuclear factor kappa B
ligand (RANKL) inhibitor
GENERAL USES:
Osteoporosis,
postmenopausal
osteoporosis, bone
tumors
DOSAGE FORMS:
Injection: 60 mg, 120 mg

DESIPRAMINE
des IP ra meen
TRADE NAME(S):
Norpramin
THERAPEUTIC CLASS:
Antidepressant
GENERAL USES:
Depression
DOSAGE FORMS:
Tablets: 10 mg, 25 mg,
50 mg, 75 mg, 100 mg,
150 mg

DESLORATADINE
des lor AT a deen
TRADE NAME(S):
Clarinex, Clarinex
Redi-tabs
THERAPEUTIC CLASS:
Antihistamine
GENERAL USES:
Allergic rhinitis, chronic
urticaria
DOSAGE FORMS:
Tablets: 5 mg; Orally
disintegrating tablets:
2.5 mg, 5 mg; Syrup:
0.5 mg/mL

DESLORATADINE/
PSEUDOEPHEDRINE
des lor AT a deen/soo doe e
FED rin
TRADE NAME(S):
Clarinex-D 12 hour,
Clarinex-D 24 hour
THERAPEUTIC CLASS:
Antihistamine/decongestant
GENERAL USES:
Seasonal allergic rhinitis
DOSAGE FORMS:
Tablets (various release):
2.5 mg/120 mg, 5 mg/
240 mg

DESONIDE
DES oh nide
TRADE NAME(S):
DesOwen, Tridesilon,
Verdeso

THERAPEUTIC CLASS:
Corticosteroid (topical)
GENERAL USES:
Various skin conditions
DOSAGE FORMS:
Ointment, Cream, Foam, and Lotion: 0.05%

DESOXIMETASONE
dess OKS ee MET ah sone
TRADE NAME(S):
Topicort
THERAPEUTIC CLASS:
Anti-psoriasis agent
GENERAL USES:
Plaque psoriasis
DOSAGE FORMS:
Topical spray: 0.25%

DESVENLAFAXINE
des VEN la FAX een
TRADE NAME(S):
Khedezla, Pristiq
THERAPEUTIC CLASS:
Antidepressant
GENERAL USES:
Depression
DOSAGE FORMS:
Tablets: 50 mg, 100 mg; Extended-release tablets: 50 mg, 100 mg

DEXAMETHASONE (INTRAVITREAL IMPLANT)
deks a METH a sone
TRADE NAME(S):
Ozurdex

THERAPEUTIC CLASS:
Glucocorticoid
GENERAL USES:
Macular edema related to BRVO/CRVO
DOSAGE FORMS:
Intravitreal implant: 0.7 mg

DEXAMETHASONE (OCULAR)
deks a METH a sone
TRADE NAME(S):
AK-Dex, Maxidex
THERAPEUTIC CLASS:
Ocular agent (steroid)
GENERAL USES:
Ocular inflammation
DOSAGE FORMS:
Ophthalmic solution, Suspension, Ointment: 0.1%

DEXAMETHASONE (ORAL)
deks a METH a sone
TRADE NAME(S):
Decadron, Dexone, Hexadrol
THERAPEUTIC CLASS:
Glucocorticoid
GENERAL USES:
Endocrine, skin, blood disorders
DOSAGE FORMS:
Tablets: 0.25 mg, 0.5 mg, 0.75 mg, 1 mg, 1.5 mg, 2 mg, 4 mg, 6 mg; Elixir and Solution: 0.5 mg/

5 mL; Concentrated
solution: 1 mg/1 mL

**DEXAMETHASONE
ACETATE**
deks a METH a sone
TRADE NAME(S):
Dalalone LA, Decadron LA
THERAPEUTIC CLASS:
Glucocorticoid
GENERAL USES:
Endocrine, skin, blood
disorders
DOSAGE FORMS:
Injection: 8 mg, 16 mg,
40 mg, 80 mg

**DEXAMETHASONE
SODIUM PHOSPHATE**
deks a METH a sone
TRADE NAME(S):
Dalalone, Decadron
Phosphate, Dexasone
THERAPEUTIC CLASS:
Glucocorticoid
GENERAL USES:
Endocrine, skin, blood
disorders
DOSAGE FORMS:
Injection: 4 mg, 10 mg,
20 mg, 40 mg, 100 mg,
120 mg, 240 mg

DEXLANSOPRAZOLE
DEX lan SOE pra zole
TRADE NAME(S):
Dexilant

THERAPEUTIC CLASS:
Gastric acid secretion
inhbiitor
GENERAL USES:
Erosive esophagitis, GERD
DOSAGE FORMS:
Delayed-release capsules:
30 mg, 60 mg

DEXMETHYLPHENIDATE
deks meth il FEN i date
TRADE NAME(S):
Focalin, Focalin XR
THERAPEUTIC CLASS:
CNS stimulant
GENERAL USES:
ADHD
DOSAGE FORMS:
Tablets: 2.5 mg, 5 mg,
10 mg; Extended-release
capsules: 5 mg, 10 mg,
20 mg

**DEXTROAMPHETAMINE
SULFATE**
deks troe am FET a meen
TRADE NAME(S):
Dexedrine
THERAPEUTIC CLASS:
Amphetamine
GENERAL USES:
Obesity
DOSAGE FORMS:
Tablets: 5 mg, 10 mg;
Sustained-release
capsules: 5 mg, 10 mg,
15 mg; Elixir:
5 mg/5 mL

DEXTROAMPHETAMINE/ AMPHETAMINE

deks troe am FET a meen/am FET a meen

Trade Name(s):
Adderall, Adderall XR

Therapeutic Class:
Amphetamine

General Uses:
ADHD

Dosage Forms:
Tablets: 5 mg, 10 mg, 20 mg, 30 mg; Extended-release capsules: 10 mg, 20 mg, 30 mg

DEXTROMETHORPHAN HYDROBROMIDE/ QUINIDINE SULFATE

DEX troe meth OR fan HYE droe BROE mide/KWIN i deen SUL fate

Trade Name(s):
Nuedexta

Therapeutic Class:
Psychiatric agent

General Uses:
Emotional lability with ALS or MS

Dosage Forms:
Capsules: 20 mg/10 mg

DIAZEPAM

dye AZ e pam

Trade Name(s):
Valium

Therapeutic Class:
Antianxiety agent, anticonvulsant, muscle relaxant

General Uses:
Anxiety, alcohol withdrawal, seizures, muscle relaxant

Dosage Forms:
Tablets: 2 mg, 5 mg, 10 mg; Solution: 5 mg/ 5 mL, 5 mg/mL; Injection: 10 mg, 50 mg

DICLOFENAC (OCULAR)

dye KLOE fen ak

Trade Name(s):
Voltaren

Therapeutic Class:
Ocular agent

General Uses:
Postoperative ocular inflammation

Dosage Forms:
Ophthalmic solution: 0.1%

DICLOFENAC (ORAL)

dye KLOE fen ak

Trade Name(s):
Cambia, Cataflam, Voltaren, Voltaren-XR, Zipsor, Zorvolex

Therapeutic Class:
Anti-inflammatory/ analgesic

General Uses:
Osteoarthritis, rheumatoid arthritis, pain

DOSAGE FORMS:
Capsules: 18 mg, 25 mg,
35 mg; Tablets
and Delayed-release
tablets: 25 mg,
50 mg, 75 mg; Extended-
release tablets: 100 mg;
Solution (oral): 50 mg

DICLOFENAC EPOLAMINE (TRANSDERMAL)
dye KLOE fen ak
TRADE NAME(S):
Flector
THERAPEUTIC CLASS:
Anti-inflammatory/
analgesic
GENERAL USES:
Acute pain
DOSAGE FORMS:
Patch: 180 mg

DICLOFENAC SODIUM (TOPICAL)
dye KLOE fen ak
TRADE NAME(S):
Pennsaid, Voltaren Gel
THERAPEUTIC CLASS:
Anti-inflammatory,
analgesic
GENERAL USES:
Osteoarthritis (knee,
hand)
DOSAGE FORMS:
Solution (topical): 1.5%,
2%; Gel: 1%

DICLOFENAC/ MISOPROSTOL
dye KLOE fen ak/mye soe
PROST ole
TRADE NAME(S):
Arthrotec
THERAPEUTIC CLASS:
Analgesic/GI protectant
GENERAL USES:
Arthritis
DOSAGE FORMS:
Tablets: 50 mg/200 mcg,
75 mg/200 mcg

DICLOXACILLIN
dye kloks a SIL in
TRADE NAME(S):
Dynapen, Dycill, Pathocil
THERAPEUTIC CLASS:
Anti-infective
GENERAL USES:
Bacterial infections
DOSAGE FORMS:
Capsules: 125 mg,
250 mg, 500 mg;
Suspension: 62.5 mg/
5 mL

DICYCLOMINE
dye SYE kloe meen
TRADE NAME(S):
Bentyl, Byclomine,
Di-Spaz
THERAPEUTIC CLASS:
GI antispasmodic
GENERAL USES:
Irritable bowel syndrome

Dosage Forms:
Capsules: 10 mg, 20 mg;
Tablets: 20 mg; Syrup:
10 mg/5 mL

DIDANOSINE (ddl)
dye DAN oh seen
Trade Name(s):
Videx, Videx EC
Therapeutic Class:
Antiviral
General Uses:
HIV infection
Dosage Forms:
Chewable tablets: 25 mg,
50 mg, 100 mg, 150 mg,
200 mg; Powder: 100 mg,
167 mg, 250 mg, 375 mg,
2 g, 4 g; Delayed-release
capsules: 125 mg,
200 mg, 250 mg,
400 mg

DIFLUNISAL
dye FLOO ni sal
Trade Name(s):
Dolobid
Therapeutic Class:
Anti-inflammatory/
analgesic
General Uses:
Pain, osteoarthritis,
rheumatoid arthritis
Dosage Forms:
Tablets: 250 mg, 500 mg

DIFLUPREDNATE (OCULAR)
DYE floo PRED nate
Trade Name(s):
Durezol
Therapeutic Class:
Corticosteroid (ocular)
General Uses:
Surgically induced ocular
inflammation and pain
Dosage Forms:
Ophthalmic solution:
0.05%

DIGOXIN
di JOKS in
Trade Name(s):
Lanoxicaps, Lanoxin,
Digitek
Therapeutic Class:
Cardiac agent
General Uses:
CHF, atrial fibrillation
Dosage Forms:
Capsules: 0.05 mg,
0.1 mg, 0.2 mg; Tablets:
0.125 mg, 0.25 mg; Elixir:
0.05 mg/mL; Injection:
0.1 mg, 0.25 mg, 0.5 mg

DIHYDROERGOTAMINE
dye hye droe er GOT a meen
Trade Name(s):
Migranal
Therapeutic Class:
Anti-migraine agent
General Uses:
Migraines

DOSAGE FORMS:
Nasal spray: 4 mg/mL

DILTIAZEM
dil TYE a zem
TRADE NAME(S):
Cardizem CD,
Cardizem LA,
Dilacor XR, Tiazac,
Taztia XT
THERAPEUTIC CLASS:
Antihypertensive,
antianginal
GENERAL USES:
Hypertension, angina
DOSAGE FORMS:
Tablets: 30 mg, 60 mg,
90 mg, 120 mg;
Extended-release
capsules and tablets:
120 mg, 180 mg, 240 mg,
300 mg, 360 mg, 420 mg;
Injection: 25 mg, 50 mg,
125 mg

DILTIAZEM/ENALAPRIL
dil TYE a zem/e NAL a pril
TRADE NAME(S):
Teczem
THERAPEUTIC CLASS:
Antihypertensive
GENERAL USES:
Hypertension
DOSAGE FORMS:
Extended-release tablets:
180 mg/5 mg

DIMENHYDRINATE
dye men HYE drih nate
TRADE NAME(S):
Dramamine, Driminate
THERAPEUTIC CLASS:
Antiemetic/antivertigo
agent
GENERAL USES:
Motion sickness
DOSAGE FORMS:
Tablets: 50 mg

DIMETHYL FUMARATE
dye METH il
TRADE NAME(S):
Tecfidera
THERAPEUTIC CLASS:
MS agent
GENERAL USES:
MS
DOSAGE FORMS:
Delayed-release capsules:
120 mg, 240 mg

DIPHENHYDRAMINE
dye fen HYE dra meen
TRADE NAME(S):
Benadryl, Diphen,
Sominex,
Unisom SleepGels
THERAPEUTIC CLASS:
Antihistamine, antiemetic
GENERAL USES:
Pruritus, allergies, sleep
aid, cough aid
DOSAGE FORMS:
Tablets and Capsules:

25 mg, 50 mg; Chewable
tablets: 12.5 mg; Liquid,
Solution, Elixir, and
Syrup: 12.5 mg/5 mL;
Cream: 1%, 2%

DIPIVEFRIN
dye PI ve frin
TRADE NAME(S):
Propine, AKPro
THERAPEUTIC CLASS:
Ocular agent
GENERAL USES:
Glaucoma
DOSAGE FORMS:
Ophthalmic solution: 0.1%

DIPYRIDAMOLE
dye peer ID a mole
TRADE NAME(S):
Persantine
THERAPEUTIC CLASS:
Antiplatelet agent
GENERAL USES:
Preventive therapy for
blood clots
DOSAGE FORMS:
Tablets: 25 mg, 50 mg,
75 mg

DIRITHROMYCIN
dye RITH roe mye sin
TRADE NAME(S):
Dynabac
THERAPEUTIC CLASS:
Anti-infective

GENERAL USES:
Bacterial infections
DOSAGE FORMS:
Tablets: 250 mg

DISOPYRAMIDE
dye soe PEER a mide
TRADE NAME(S):
Norpace, Norpace CR
THERAPEUTIC CLASS:
Antiarrhythmic
GENERAL USES:
Ventricular
arrhythmias
DOSAGE FORMS:
Capsules and Extended-
release capsules: 100 mg,
150 mg

DISULFIRAM
dye SUL fi ram
TRADE NAME(S):
Antabuse
THERAPEUTIC CLASS:
Antialcoholic
GENERAL USES:
Alcohol abstinence
DOSAGE FORMS:
Tablets: 250 mg, 500 mg

DOBUTAMINE
doe BYOO ta meen
TRADE NAME(S):
Dobutrex
THERAPEUTIC CLASS:
Cardiac agent
GENERAL USES:
Increases cardiac

contractility

DOSAGE FORMS:
Injection: 250 mg

DOCETAXEL
DOE se TAX el

TRADE NAME(S):
Docefrez, Taxotere

THERAPEUTIC CLASS:
Antineoplastic

GENERAL USES:
Various cancers

DOSAGE FORMS:
Injection: 20 mg, 80 mg,
130 mg, 140 mg, 200 mg

DOCOSANOL
doe KOE san ole

TRADE NAME(S):
Abreva

THERAPEUTIC CLASS:
Antiviral

GENERAL USES:
Treatment of fever blisters,
cold sores

DOSAGE FORMS:
Cream: 10%

DOFETILIDE
doe FET il ide

TRADE NAME(S):
Tikosyn

THERAPEUTIC CLASS:
Antiarrhythmic

GENERAL USES:
Atrial fibrillation/flutter

DOSAGE FORMS:
Capsules: 125 mcg,
250 mcg, 500 mcg

DOLASETRON
dol A se tron

TRADE NAME(S):
Anzemet

THERAPEUTIC CLASS:
Antiemetic

GENERAL USES:
Surgical or chemotherapy
nausea/vomiting

DOSAGE FORMS:
Tablets: 50 mg, 100 mg;
Injection: 12.5 mg,
100 mg

DOLUTEGRAVIR
DOE loo TEG ra veer

TRADE NAME(S):
Tivicay

THERAPEUTIC CLASS:
Antiviral

GENERAL USES:
HIV infection

DOSAGE FORMS:
Tablets: 50 mg

DONEPEZIL
doh NEP e zil

TRADE NAME(S):
Aricept, Aricept ODT

THERAPEUTIC CLASS:
Alzheimer's agent

GENERAL USES:
Alzheimer's disease

DOSAGE FORMS:
Orally disintegrating
tablets and Tablets: 5 mg,
10 mg; Tablets: 23 mg

DOPAMINE
DOE pa meen
TRADE NAME(S):
Intropin
THERAPEUTIC CLASS:
Cardiac agent
GENERAL USES:
Increases cardiac output
DOSAGE FORMS:
Injection: 200 mg,
400 mg, 800 mg, 1.6 g

DORIPENEM
dore i PEN em
TRADE NAME(S):
Doribax
THERAPEUTIC CLASS:
Anti-infective
GENERAL USES:
Bacterial infection
DOSAGE FORMS:
Injection: 500 mg

DORZOLAMIDE
dor ZOLE a mide
TRADE NAME(S):
Trusopt
THERAPEUTIC CLASS:
Ocular agent
GENERAL USES:
Glaucoma/ocular
hypertension
DOSAGE FORMS:
Ophthalmic solution: 2%

DORZOLAMIDE/ TIMOLOL
dor ZOLE a mide/TYE moe
lole
TRADE NAME(S):
Cosopt, Cosopt PF
THERAPEUTIC CLASS:
Ocular agent
GENERAL USES:
Glaucoma, ocular
hypertension
DOSAGE FORMS:
Ophthalmic solution:
2%/0.5%

DOXAZOSIN
doks AY zoe sin
TRADE NAME(S):
Cardura
THERAPEUTIC CLASS:
Antihypertensive, BPH
agent
GENERAL USES:
Hypertension, BPH
DOSAGE FORMS:
Tablets: 1 mg, 2 mg,
4 mg, 8 mg

DOXEPIN (ORAL)
DOKS e pin
TRADE NAME(S):
Sinequan, Silenor
THERAPEUTIC CLASS:
Antidepressant, hypnotic
GENERAL USES:
Depression, insomnia

DOSAGE FORMS:
Capsules: 10 mg, 25 mg,
50 mg, 75 mg, 100 mg,
150 mg; Solution:
10 mg/mL; Tablets: 3 mg,
6 mg

DOXEPIN (TOPICAL)
DOKS e pin
TRADE NAME(S):
Zonalon
THERAPEUTIC CLASS:
Antipruritic (topical)
GENERAL USES:
Pruritus
DOSAGE FORMS:
Cream: 5%

DOXYCYCLINE
doks i SYE kleen
TRADE NAME(S):
Vibramycin,
Vibra-Tabs,
Doxy, Doxychel, Acticlate
THERAPEUTIC CLASS:
Anti-infective
GENERAL USES:
Bacterial infections
DOSAGE FORMS:
Capsules: 20 mg, 50 mg,
75 mg, 100 mg, 150 mg;
Tablets: 50 mg, 100 mg;
Suspension: 25 mg/5 mL;
Syrup: 50 mg/5 mL

DOXYCYCLINE
doks i SYE kleen
TRADE NAME(S):
Oracea
THERAPEUTIC CLASS:
Anti-infective
GENERAL USES:
Rosacea lesions
DOSAGE FORMS:
Capsules: 40 mg

DOXYCYCLINE
doks i SYE kleen
TRADE NAME(S):
Atridox
THERAPEUTIC CLASS:
Anti-infective
GENERAL USES:
Periodontitis
DOSAGE FORMS:
Oral gel: 10%

DOXYLAMINE SUCCINATE/ PYRIDOXINE HCL
doks IL a meen/peer ih
DOKS een
TRADE NAME(S):
Diclegis
THERAPEUTIC CLASS:
Antihistamine/vitamin B6
analog
GENERAL USES:
Nausea/vomiting in
pregnancy
DOSAGE FORMS:
Delayed-release tablets:
10 mg/10 mg

DRONABINOL
droe NAB i nol

TRADE NAME(S):
Marinol

THERAPEUTIC CLASS:
Antiemetic

GENERAL USES:
Chemotherapy nausea/
vomiting, appetite
stimulant

DOSAGE FORMS:
Capsules: 2.5 mg, 5 mg,
10 mg

DRONEDARONE
DROE NE da rone

TRADE NAME(S):
Multaq

THERAPEUTIC CLASS:
Antiarrhythmic

GENERAL USES:
Atrial fibrillation and
flutter

DOSAGE FORMS:
Tablets: 400 mg

DROTRECOGIN ALFA
dro TRE coe jin AL fa

TRADE NAME(S):
Xigris

THERAPEUTIC CLASS:
Biological

GENERAL USES:
Sepsis

DOSAGE FORMS:
Injection: 5 mg, 20 mg

DROXIDOPA
DROKS i DOP a

TRADE NAME(S):
Northera

THERAPEUTIC CLASS:
Adrenergic,
sympathomimetic

GENERAL USES:
Dizziness,
lightheadedness

DOSAGE FORMS:
Capsules: 100 mg, 200
mg, 300 mg

DULOXETINE
doo LOKS e teen

TRADE NAME(S):
Cymbalta

THERAPEUTIC CLASS:
Antidepressant

GENERAL USES:
Depression, anxiety,
fibromyalgia

DOSAGE FORMS:
Delayed-release
capsules: 20 mg, 30 mg,
60 mg

DUTASTERIDE
doo TAS teer ide

TRADE NAME(S):
Avodart

THERAPEUTIC CLASS:
Antiandrogen

GENERAL USES:
BPH

DOSAGE FORMS:
Capsules: 0.5 mg

**DUTASTERIDE/
TAMSULOSIN**
doo TAS teer ide/tam SOO
loe sin
TRADE NAME(S):
 Jalyn
THERAPEUTIC CLASS:
 Antiandrogen/urologic
 agent
GENERAL USES:
 BPH
DOSAGE FORMS:
 Capsules: 0.5 mg/0.4 mg

ECALLANTIDE
e KAL lan tide
TRADE NAME(S):
 Kalbitor
THERAPEUTIC CLASS:
 Hematological agent
GENERAL USES:
 Hereditary angioedema
DOSAGE FORMS:
 Injection: 10 mg

ECONAZOLE
e KONE a zole
TRADE NAME(S):
 Spectazole, Ecoza
THERAPEUTIC CLASS:
 Antifungal (topical)
GENERAL USES:
 Athlete's foot, jock itch,
 ringworm
DOSAGE FORMS:
 Cream: 1%; Foam: 1%

ECULIZUMAB
e kue LIZ oo mab
TRADE NAME(S):
 Soliris
THERAPEUTIC CLASS:
 Complement inhibitor
GENERAL USES:
 Nocturnal
 hemoglobinuria
DOSAGE FORMS:
 Injection: 300 mg

EFALIZUMAB
e fa li ZOO mab
TRADE NAME(S):
 Raptiva
THERAPEUTIC CLASS:
 Immunosuppressant
GENERAL USES:
 Psoriasis
DOSAGE FORMS:
 Injection: 125 mg

EFAVIRENZ
e FAV e renz
TRADE NAME(S):
 Sustiva
THERAPEUTIC CLASS:
 Antiviral
GENERAL USES:
 HIV infection
DOSAGE FORMS:
 Capsules: 50 mg, 100 mg,
 200 mg, 600 mg; Tablets:
 200 mg

**EFAVIRENZ/
EMTRICITABINE/
TENOFOVIR
DISOPROXIL FUMARATE**
e FAV e renz/em trye SYE ta
been/te NOE fo veer
TRADE NAME(S):
Atripla
THERAPEUTIC CLASS:
Antiviral
GENERAL USES:
HIV infection
DOSAGE FORMS:
Tablets: 600 mg/200 mg/
300 mg

EFINACONAZOLE
ef in a KON a zole
TRADE NAME(S):
Jublia
THERAPEUTIC CLASS:
Antifungal
GENERAL USES:
Toenail fungal infections
DOSAGE FORMS:
Solution: 10%

ELETRIPTAN
el e TRIP tan
TRADE NAME(S):
Relpax
THERAPEUTIC CLASS:
Antimigraine
GENERAL USES:
Migraines
DOSAGE FORMS:
Tablets: 20 mg, 40 mg

ELIGLUSTAT
el i GLOO stat
TRADE NAME(S):
Cerdelga
THERAPEUTIC CLASS:
Endocrine-metabolic
agent
GENERAL USES:
Gaucher disease
DOSAGE FORMS:
Capsules: 84 mg

ELOSULFASE ALFA
EL oh SUL fase AL fa
TRADE NAME(S):
Vimizim
THERAPEUTIC CLASS:
Enzyme
GENERAL USES:
Mucopolysaccharidosis
type IV A
DOSAGE FORMS:
Injection: 5 mg

**ELTROMBOPAG
OLAMINE**
el TROM boe pag
TRADE NAME(S):
Promacta
THERAPEUTIC CLASS:
Hematological agent
GENERAL USES:
Thrombocytopenia
DOSAGE FORMS:
Tablets:
25 mg, 50 mg, 75 mg

ELVITEGRAVIR
el vi TEG ra veer
Trade Name(s):
Vitekta
Therapeutic Class:
Antiviral
General Class:
HIV infection
DOSAGE FORMS:
Tablets: 85 mg, 150 mg

ELVITEGRAVIR/ COBICISTAT/EMTRI- CITABINE/TENOFOVIR DISOPROXIL FUMARATE
EL vi TEG ra veer/koe BIK i stat/em trye SYE ta been/ten OF oh veer
Trade Name(s):
Stribild
Therapeutic Class:
Antiviral
General Uses:
HIV infection
Dosage Forms:
Tablets: 150 mg/150 mg/ 200 mg/300 mg

EMEDASTINE
em e DAS teen
Trade Name(s):
Emadine
Therapeutic Class:
Ocular agent
General Uses:
Allergic conjunctivitis

Dosage Forms:
Ophthalmic solution: 0.05%

EMPAGLIFLOZIN
EM pa gli FLOE zin
Trade Name(s):
Jardiance
Therapeutic Class:
Antidiabetic
General Class:
Diabetes (type 2)
Dosage Forms:
Tablets: 10 mg, 25 mg

EMTRICITABINE
em trye SYE ta been
Trade Name(s):
Emtriva
Therapeutic Class:
Antiviral
General Uses:
HIV infection
Dosage Forms:
Capsules: 200 mg; Solution: 10 mg/mL

EMTRICITABINE/ RILPIVIRINE/ TENOFOVIR DISOPROXIL FUMARATE
em trye SYE ta been/RIL pi VEER een/ten OF oh veer
Trade Name(s):
Complera
Therapeutic Class:
Antiviral

GENERAL USES:
HIV infection
DOSAGE FORMS:
Tablets: 200 mg/25 mg/
300 mg

ENALAPRIL
e NAL a pril
TRADE NAME(S):
Epaned, Vasotec, Vasotec IV
THERAPEUTIC CLASS:
Antihypertensive, cardiac
agent
GENERAL USES:
Hypertension, heart
failure, left ventricular
dysfunction
DOSAGE FORMS:
Tablets: 2.5 mg, 5 mg,
10 mg, 20 mg; Injection:
1.25 mg, 2.5 mg
(enalaprilat); Solution:
1 mg/mL

ENALAPRIL/HCTZ
e NAL a pril/hye droe klor oh
THYE a zide
TRADE NAME(S):
Vaseretic
THERAPEUTIC CLASS:
Antihypertensive/
diuretic
GENERAL USES:
Hypertension
DOSAGE FORMS:
Tablets: 5 mg/12.5 mg,
10 mg/25 mg

ENFUVIRTIDE
en FYOO veer tide
TRADE NAME(S):
Fuzeon
THERAPEUTIC CLASS:
Antiviral
GENERAL USES:
HIV infection
DOSAGE FORMS:
Injection: 90 mg

ENOXACIN
en OKS a sin
TRADE NAME(S):
Penetrex
THERAPEUTIC CLASS:
Anti-infective
GENERAL USES:
Bacterial infections
DOSAGE FORMS:
Tablets: 200 mg, 400 mg

ENOXAPARIN SODIUM
ee noks a PA rin
TRADE NAME(S):
Lovenox
THERAPEUTIC CLASS:
Anticoagulant (LMWH)
GENERAL USES:
Prevent blood clots
DOSAGE FORMS:
Injection: 30 mg, 40 mg,
60 mg, 80 mg, 90 mg,
100 mg, 120 mg, 150 mg

ENTACAPONE
en TA ka pone
TRADE NAME(S):
  Comtan
THERAPEUTIC CLASS:
  Antiparkinson agent
GENERAL USES:
  Parkinson's disease
DOSAGE FORMS:
  Tablets: 200 mg

ENTECAVIR
en TE ka veer
TRADE NAME(S):
  Baraclude
THERAPEUTIC CLASS:
  Antiviral
GENERAL USES:
  Chronic hepatitis B
DOSAGE FORMS:
  Solution: 0.05 mg/mL;
  Tablets: 0.5 mg, 1 mg

ENZALUTAMIDE
EN za LOO ta mide
TRADE NAME(S):
  Xtandi
THERAPEUTIC CLASS:
  Antineoplastic
GENERAL USES:
  Metastatic castration-
  resistant prostate cancer
DOSAGE FORMS:
  Capsules: 40 mg

EPINASTINE (OCULAR)
ep i NAS teen
TRADE NAME(S):
  Elestat
THERAPEUTIC CLASS:
  Ocular (antihistamine)
GENERAL USES:
  Allergic conjunctivitis
DOSAGE FORMS:
  Ophthalmic solution:
  0.05%

**EPINEPHRINE
(OPHTHALMIC)**
ep i NEF rin
TRADE NAME(S):
  Epifrin, Glaucon
THERAPEUTIC CLASS:
  Ocular agent
GENERAL USES:
  Glaucoma
DOSAGE FORMS:
  Ophthalmic solution:
  0.1%, 0.5%, 1%, 2%

EPINEPHRINE
EP i NEF rin
TRADE NAME(S):
  Adrenaclick, Adrenalin,
  Auvi-Q, Epipen, Twinject
THERAPEUTIC CLASS:
  Sympathomimetic
GENERAL USES:
  Allergic reactions, eye
  surgery
DOSAGE FORMS:
  Injection: 0.15 mg, 0.3
  mg, 1 mg, 30 mg

EPLERENONE
e PLER en one
TRADE NAME(S):
Inspra
THERAPEUTIC CLASS:
Antihypertensive
GENERAL USES:
Hypertension
DOSAGE FORMS:
Tablets: 25 mg, 50 mg, 100 mg

EPOETIN ALFA
e POE e tin
TRADE NAME(S):
Epogen, Procrit
THERAPEUTIC CLASS:
Hematological agent
GENERAL USES:
Anemia with chronic renal failure, cancer, or HIV infection
DOSAGE FORMS:
Injection: 2000 units, 3000 units, 4000 units, 10,000 units, 20,000 units

EPOPROSTENOL
E poe PROS te nol
TRADE NAME(S):
Flolan, Veletri
THERAPEUTIC CLASS:
Antihypertensive
GENERAL USES:
Pulmonary hypertension
DOSAGE FORMS:
Injection: 0.5 mg, 1.5 mg

ERGOTAMINE TARTRATE
er GOT a meen
TRADE NAME(S):
Ergomar
THERAPEUTIC CLASS:
Antimigraine agent
GENERAL USES:
Migraines
DOSAGE FORMS:
Sublingual tablets: 2 mg

ERIBULIN MESYLATE
ER i BUE lin MES i late
TRADE NAME(S):
Halaven
THERAPEUTIC CLASS:
Antineoplastic
GENERAL USES:
Metastatic breast cancer
DOSAGE FORMS:
Injection: 1 mg

ERLOTINIB
er LOE tye nib
TRADE NAME(S):
Tarceva
THERAPEUTIC CLASS:
EGFR inhibitor
GENERAL USES:
Non-small-cell lung cancer, pancreatic cancer
DOSAGE FORMS:
Tablets: 25 mg, 100 mg, 150 mg

ERTAPENEM
er ta PEN em
TRADE NAME(S):
   Invanz
THERAPEUTIC CLASS:
   Anti-infective
GENERAL USES:
   Bacterial infections
DOSAGE FORMS:
   Injection: 1 g

ERYTHROMYCIN (BASE)
er ith roe MYE sin
TRADE NAME(S):
   E-Mycin, E-Base, PCE,
   Ery-Tab, Eryc
THERAPEUTIC CLASS:
   Anti-infective
GENERAL USES:
   Bacterial infections
DOSAGE FORMS:
   Tablets: 250 mg, 333 mg,
   500 mg; Delayed-release
   capsules: 250 mg

**ERYTHROMYCIN
(OCULAR)**
er ith roe MYE sin
TRADE NAME(S):
   Ilotycin
THERAPEUTIC CLASS:
   Ocular agent
   (anti-infective)
GENERAL USES:
   Ocular infections
DOSAGE FORMS:
   Ophthalmic ointment:
   5%

**ERYTHROMYCIN
(TOPICAL)**
er ith roe MYE sin
TRADE NAME(S):
   Akne-mycin, Emgel,
   Erygel
THERAPEUTIC CLASS:
   Anti-infective (topical)
GENERAL USES:
   Acne
DOSAGE FORMS:
   Ointment and Gel: 2%;
   Solution: 1.5%, 2%

**ERYTHROMYCIN
ESTOLATE**
er ith roe MYE sin
TRADE NAME(S):
   Ilosone
THERAPEUTIC CLASS:
   Anti-infective
GENERAL USES:
   Bacterial infections
DOSAGE FORMS:
   Tablets: 500 mg;
   Capsules: 250 mg;
   Suspension: 125 mg/
   5 mL, 250 mg/5 mL

**ERYTHROMYCIN
ETHYLSUCCINATE**
er ith roe MYE sin
TRADE NAME(S):
   EryPed, EES
THERAPEUTIC CLASS:
   Anti-infective
GENERAL USES:
   Bacterial infections

DOSAGE FORMS:
Tablets: 400 mg;
Chewable tablets:
200 mg; Suspension:
200 mg/5 mL, 400 mg/
5 mL, 100 mg/2.5 mL

ERYTHROMYCIN LACTOBIONATE
er ith roe MYE sin
TRADE NAME(S):
Erythrocin
THERAPEUTIC CLASS:
Anti-infective
GENERAL USES:
Bacterial infections
DOSAGE FORMS:
Injection: 500 mg, 1 g

ERYTHROMYCIN STEARATE
er ith roe MYE sin
TRADE NAME(S):
Erythrocin
THERAPEUTIC CLASS:
Anti-infective
GENERAL USES:
Bacterial infections
DOSAGE FORMS:
Tablets: 250 mg, 500 mg

ERYTHROMYCIN/ BENZOYL PEROXIDE
er ith roe MYE sin/BEN zoyl
per OKS ide
TRADE NAME(S):
Benzamycin
THERAPEUTIC CLASS:
Anti-infective (topical)

GENERAL USES:
Acne
DOSAGE FORMS:
Gel: 30 mg/50 mg per g

ESCITALOPRAM
es sye TAL oh pram
TRADE NAME(S):
Lexapro
THERAPEUTIC CLASS:
Antidepressant
GENERAL USES:
Depression, anxiety
DOSAGE FORMS:
Tablets: 5 mg, 10 mg,
20 mg; Solution: 1 mg/mL

ESLICARBAZEPINE ACETATE
ES li kar BAZ e peen
TRADE NAME(S):
Aptiom
THERAPEUTIC CLASS:
Anticonvulsant
GENERAL USES:
Partial seizures
DOSAGE FORMS:
Tablets: 200 mg, 400 mg,
600 mg, 800 mg

ESOMEPRAZOLE
es oh ME pray zol
TRADE NAME(S):
Nexium
THERAPEUTIC CLASS:
Gastric acid secretion
inhibitor

GENERAL USES:
GERD, erosive
esophagitis, Zollinger-
Ellison syndrome, NSAID-
associated ulcer

DOSAGE FORMS:
Injection and
Capsules:
20 mg, 40 mg

ESOMEPRAZOLE/ NAPROXEN
es oh ME pray zol/ na
PROKS en

TRADE NAME(S):
Vimovo

THERAPEUTIC CLASS:
Gastric acid secretion
inhibitor/NSAID

GENERAL USES:
Osteoarthritis, rheumatoid
arthritis, ankylosing
spondylitis

DOSAGE FORMS:
Tablets: 20 mg/375 mg,
20 mg/500 mg

ESTAZOLAM
es TA zoe lam

TRADE NAME(S):
ProSom

THERAPEUTIC CLASS:
Sedative/hypnotic

GENERAL USES:
Insomnia

DOSAGE FORMS:
Tablets: 1 mg, 2 mg

ESTRADIOL (GEL)
es tra DYE ole

TRADE NAME(S):
EstroGel, Divigel

THERAPEUTIC CLASS:
Hormone (estrogen)

GENERAL USES:
Vasomotor symptoms of
menopause

DOSAGE FORMS:
Gel/Pump: 0.06%; Gel:
0.1%

ESTRADIOL (SPRAY)
es tra DYE ole

TRADE NAME(S):
Evamist

THERAPEUTIC CLASS:
Hormone (estrogen)

GENERAL USES:
Estrogen replacement

DOSAGE FORMS:
Spray: 1.53 mg/spray

ESTRADIOL (TRANSDERMAL)
es tra DYE ole

TRADE NAME(S):
FemPatch, Vivelle, Alora,
Estraderm, Climara,
Menostar, Vivelle-Dot,
Minivelle

THERAPEUTIC CLASS:
Hormone (estrogen)

GENERAL USES:
Estrogen replacement

DOSAGE FORMS:
Transdermal patch

(release rate/24 hr):
0.014 mg, 0.025 mg,
0.0375 mg, 0.05 mg,
0.075 mg, 0.1 mg

ESTRADIOL
(VAGINAL RING)
es tra DYE ole
TRADE NAME(S):
Femring
THERAPEUTIC CLASS:
Hormone (estrogen)
GENERAL USES:
Vasomotor symptoms of
menopause
DOSAGE FORMS:
Vaginal ring: 0.05 mg/day,
0.1 mg/day

ESTRADIOL, 17-BETA
(TOPICAL EMULSION)
es tra DYE ole
TRADE NAME(S):
Estrasorb
THERAPEUTIC CLASS:
Hormone (estrogen)
GENERAL USES:
Estrogen replacement
DOSAGE FORMS:
Topical emulsion pouch:
1.74 g (4.35 mg estradiol)

ESTRADIOL VALERATE/
DIENOGEST
ES tra dye ole/dye EN oh jest
TRADE NAME(S):
Natazia

THERAPEUTIC CLASS:
Contraceptive
GENERAL USES:
Contraception, heavy
menstrual bleeding
DOSAGE FORMS:
Tablets: Phase 1:
3 mg/0mg; Phase 2:
2 mg/2 mg; Phase 3:
2 mg/3 mg; Phase 4:
1 mg/0 mg

ESTRADIOL/
DROSPIRENONE
es tra DYE ole/droh SPYE
re none
TRADE NAME(S):
Angeliq
THERAPEUTIC CLASS:
Hormone
GENERAL USES:
Menopausal symptoms
DOSAGE FORMS:
Tablets: 0.5 mg/0.25 mg,
1 mg/0.5 mg

ESTRADIOL/
LEVONORGESTREL
(TRANSDERMAL)
es tra DYE ole/LEE voe nor
jes trel
TRADE NAME(S):
Climara Pro
THERAPEUTIC CLASS:
Hormone (estrogen/
progestin)

GENERAL USES:
Vasomotor symptoms of menopause

DOSAGE FORMS:
Patch: 45 mcg/15 mcg

ESTRADIOL/ NORETHINDRONE
es tra DYE ole/nor eth IN drone

TRADE NAME(S):
Activella

THERAPEUTIC CLASS:
Hormone (estrogen/ progestin)

GENERAL USES:
Estrogen replacement

DOSAGE FORMS:
Tablets: 1 mg/0.5 mg

ESTROGENS, CONJUGATED
ES troe jenz

TRADE NAME(S):
Premarin, Premarin IV

THERAPEUTIC CLASS:
Hormone (estrogen)

GENERAL USES:
Estrogen replacement

DOSAGE FORMS:
Tablets: 0.3 mg, 0.625 mg, 0.9 mg, 1.25 mg, 2.5 mg; Injection: 25 mg

ESTROGENS, ESTERIFIED
ES troe jenz, es TER i fied

TRADE NAME(S):
Estratab, Menest

THERAPEUTIC CLASS:
Hormone (estrogen)

GENERAL USES:
Estrogen replacement

DOSAGE FORMS:
Tablets: 0.3 mg, 0.625 mg, 1.25 mg, 2.5 mg

ESTROGENS A, CONJUGATED (SYNTHETIC)
ES troe jenz

TRADE NAME(S):
Cenestin

THERAPEUTIC CLASS:
Hormone

GENERAL USES:
Vasomotor symptoms of menopause, vaginal atrophy

DOSAGE FORMS:
Tablets: 0.3 mg, 0.625 mg, 0.9 mg, 1.25 mg

ESTROGENS B, CONJUGATED (SYNTHETIC)
ES troe jenz

TRADE NAME(S):
Enjuvia

THERAPEUTIC CLASS:
Hormone

GENERAL USES:
  Vasomotor symptoms of
  menopause
DOSAGE FORMS:
  Tablets: 0.625 mg, 1.25 mg

ESTROGENS, CONJUGATED/ MEDROXY- PROGESTERONE
ES troe jenz/me DROKS ee
proe JES te rone
TRADE NAME(S):
  Prempro,
  Premphase
THERAPEUTIC CLASS:
  Hormone (estrogen/
  progestin)
GENERAL USES:
  Estrogen replacement
DOSAGE FORMS:
  Tablets: 0.625 mg/5 mg,
  0.625 mg/2.5 mg,
  0.3 mg/1.5 mg, 0.45 mg/
  1.5 mg

ESTROPIPATE
ES troe pih pate
TRADE NAME(S):
  Ogen, Ortho-Est
THERAPEUTIC CLASS:
  Hormone (estrogen)
GENERAL USES:
  Estrogen replacement
DOSAGE FORMS:
  Tablets: 0.625 mg,
  1.25 mg, 2.5 mg, 5 mg;
  Vaginal cream: 0.15%

ESZOPICLONE
es zoe PIK lone
TRADE NAME(S):
  Lunesta
THERAPEUTIC CLASS:
  Hypnotic
GENERAL USES:
  Insomnia
DOSAGE FORMS:
  Tablets: 1 mg, 2 mg,
  3 mg

ETANERCEPT
et a NER sept
TRADE NAME(S):
  Enbrel
THERAPEUTIC CLASS:
  Immunomodulator
GENERAL USES:
  Rheumatoid and psoriatic
  arthritis, plaque psoriasis,
  ankylosing spondylitis
DOSAGE FORMS:
  Injection: 25 mg,
  50 mg

ETHACRYNIC ACID
eth a KRIN ik AS id
TRADE NAME(S):
  Edecrin
THERAPEUTIC CLASS:
  Diuretic
GENERAL USES:
  CHF-related edema,
  hypertension
DOSAGE FORMS:
  Tablets: 25 mg, 50 mg

ETHAMBUTOL
e THAM byoo tole
Trade Name(s):
Myambutol
Therapeutic Class:
Antituberculosis agent
General Uses:
Tuberculosis
Dosage Forms:
Tablets: 100 mg, 400 mg

ETHINYL ESTRADIOL
ETH in il es tra DYE ole
Trade Name(s):
Estinyl
Therapeutic Class:
Hormone (estrogen)
General Uses:
Estrogen replacement
Dosage Forms:
Tablets: 0.02 mg,
0.05 mg, 0.25 mg,
0.5 mg

ETHINYL ESTRADIOL/ DESOGESTREL
ETH in il es tra DYE ole/des
oh JES trel
Trade Name(s):
Desogen, Ortho-Cept,
Apri
Therapeutic Class:
Contraceptive
(monophasic)
General Uses:
Contraception
Dosage Forms:
Tablets: 30 mcg/0.15 mg

ETHINYL ESTRADIOL/ DESOGESTREL
ETH in il es tra DYE ole/des
oh JES trel
Trade Name(s):
Mircette, Kariva
Therapeutic Class:
Contraceptive (biphasic)
General Uses:
Contraception
Dosage Forms:
Tablets: Phase 1: 20 mcg/
0.15 mg; Phase 2: 10 mcg
(EE)

ETHINYL ESTRADIOL/ DROSPIRENONE
ETH in il es tra DYE ole/droh
SPYE re none
Trade Name(s):
Yasmin
Therapeutic Class:
Contraceptive
(monophasic)
General Uses:
Contraception
Dosage Forms:
Tablets: 0.03 mg/3 mg

ETHINYL ESTRADIOL/ DROSPIRENONE
ETH in il es tra DYE ole/droh
SPYE re none
Trade Name(s):
Yaz
Therapeutic Class:
Contraceptive

GENERAL USES:
Contraception, PMDD
DOSAGE FORMS:
Tablets: 20 mcg/3 mg

ETHINYL ESTRADIOL/ DROSPIRENONE/ LEVOMEFOLATE CALCIUM
ETH in il es tra DYE ole/droh SPYE re none/lee voe me FOE late
TRADE NAME(S):
Beyaz
THERAPEUTIC CLASS:
Contraceptive
GENERAL USES:
Contraception
DOSAGE FORMS:
Tablets: 0.02 mg/ 3 mg/0.451 mg

ETHINYL ESTRADIOL/ ETHYNODIOL
ETH in il es tra DYE ole/e thye noe DYE ole
TRADE NAME(S):
Demulen 1/50, Zovia 1/50E
THERAPEUTIC CLASS:
Contraceptive (monophasic)
GENERAL USES:
Contraception
DOSAGE FORMS:
Tablets: 50 mcg/1 mg

ETHINYL ESTRADIOL/ ETHYNODIOL
ETH in il es tra DYE ole/e thye noe DYE ole
TRADE NAME(S):
Demulen 1/35, Zovia 1/35E
THERAPEUTIC CLASS:
Contraceptive (monophasic)
GENERAL USES:
Contraception
DOSAGE FORMS:
Tablets: 35 mcg/1 mg

ETHINYL ESTRADIOL/ ETONOGESTREL
ETH in il es tra DYE ole/et oh noe JES trel
TRADE NAME(S):
NuvaRing
THERAPEUTIC CLASS:
Contraceptive
GENERAL USES:
Contraception
DOSAGE FORMS:
Vaginal ring (release rate/ 24 hr): 15 mcg/120 mcg

ETHINYL ESTRADIOL/ LEVONORGESTREL
ETH in il es tra DYE ole/LEE voe nor jes trel
TRADE NAME(S):
Preven
THERAPEUTIC CLASS:
Contraceptive (emergency)

GENERAL USES:
Emergency contraception
DOSAGE FORMS:
Tablets: 50 mcg/0.25 mg

ETHINYL ESTRADIOL/ LEVONORGESTREL
ETH in il es tra DYE ole/LEE voe nor jes trel
TRADE NAME(S):
Seasonique
THERAPEUTIC CLASS:
Contraceptive
GENERAL USES:
Contraception
DOSAGE FORMS:
Tablets: 30 mcg/15 mcg, 10 mcg/15 mcg

ETHINYL ESTRADIOL/ LEVONORGESTREL
ETH in il es tra DYE ole/LEE voe nor jes trel
TRADE NAME(S):
Levlen, Levora 0.15/30, Nordette, Portia
THERAPEUTIC CLASS:
Contraceptive (monophasic)
GENERAL USES:
Contraception
DOSAGE FORMS:
Tablets: 30 mcg/0.15 mg

ETHINYL ESTRADIOL/ LEVONORGESTREL
ETH in il es tra DYE ole/LEE voe nor jes trel
TRADE NAME(S):
Seasonale
THERAPEUTIC CLASS:
Hormone (estrogen/ progestin)
GENERAL USES:
Contraception (91-day regimen)
DOSAGE FORMS:
Tablets: 30 mcg/150 mcg

ETHINYL ESTRADIOL/ LEVONORGESTREL
ETH in il es tra DYE ole/LEE voe nor jes trel
TRADE NAME(S):
Levlite, Alesse, Lessina, Aviane
THERAPEUTIC CLASS:
Contraceptive (monophasic)
GENERAL USES:
Contraception
DOSAGE FORMS:
Tablets: 20 mcg/0.1 mg

ETHINYL ESTRADIOL/ LEVONORGESTREL
ETH in il es tra DYE ole/LEE voe nor jes trel
TRADE NAME(S):
Lybrel
THERAPEUTIC CLASS:
Contraceptive

GENERAL USES:
Contraception

DOSAGE FORMS:
Tablets: 20 mcg/90 mcg

ETHINYL ESTRADIOL/ LEVONORGESTREL

ETH in il es tra DYE ole/LEE voe nor jes trel

TRADE NAME(S):
Enpresse, Tri-Levlen, Triphasil, Trivora-28

THERAPEUTIC CLASS:
Contraceptive (triphasic)

GENERAL USES:
Contraception

DOSAGE FORMS:
Tablets: Phase 1: 30 mcg/0.05 mg; Phase 2: 40 mcg/ 0.075 mg; Phase 3: 30 mcg/ 0.125 mg

ETHINYL ESTRADIOL/ LEVONORGESTREL

ETH in il es tra DYE ole/LEE voe nor jes trel

TRADE NAME(S):
Quartette

THERAPEUTIC CLASS:
Contraceptive

GENERAL USES:
Contraception

DOSAGE FORMS:
Tablets: Phase 1: 0.02 mg/0.15 mg; Phase 2: 0.025 mg/0.15 mg; Phase 3: 0.03 mg/0.15 mg; Phase 4: 0.1 mg/0 mg

ETHINYL ESTRADIOL/ NORELGESTROMIN

ETH in il es tra DYE ole/nor el JES troe min

TRADE NAME(S):
Ortho Evra

THERAPEUTIC CLASS:
Contraceptive

GENERAL USES:
Contraception

DOSAGE FORMS:
Transdermal patch (release rate/24 hr): 20 mcg/150 mcg

ETHINYL ESTRADIOL/ NORETHINDRONE

ETH in il es tra DYE ole/nor eth IN drone

TRADE NAME(S):
Genora 1/35, Nelova 1/35E, Norethin 1/35E, Norinyl 1+35, Nortrel 1/35, Necon 1/35, Ortho-Novum 1/35

THERAPEUTIC CLASS:
Contraceptive (monophasic)

GENERAL USES:
Contraception

DOSAGE FORMS:
Tablets: 35 mcg/1 mg

ETHINYL ESTRADIOL/ NORETHINDRONE

ETH in il es tra DYE ole/nor eth IN drone

TRADE NAME(S):
Brevicon, Modicon, Genora 0.5/35, Nelova 0.5/35E, Necon 0.5/35, Nortrel 0.5/35

THERAPEUTIC CLASS:
Contraceptive (monophasic)

GENERAL USES:
Contraception

DOSAGE FORMS:
Tablets: 35 mcg/0.5 mg

ETHINYL ESTRADIOL/ NORETHINDRONE

ETH in il es tra DYE ole/nor eth IN drone

TRADE NAME(S):
Ovcon 35

THERAPEUTIC CLASS:
Contraceptive (monophasic)

GENERAL USES:
Contraception

DOSAGE FORMS:
Chewable tablets and Tablets: 35 mcg/ 0.4 mg

ETHINYL ESTRADIOL/ NORETHINDRONE

ETH in il es tra DYE ole/nor eth IN drone

TRADE NAME(S):
Loestrin 1.5/30, Microgestin 1.5/30

THERAPEUTIC CLASS:
Contraceptive (monophasic)

GENERAL USES:
Contraception

DOSAGE FORMS:
Tablets: 30 mcg/ 1.5 mg

ETHINYL ESTRADIOL/ NORETHINDRONE

ETH in il es tra DYE ole/nor eth IN drone

TRADE NAME(S):
Loestrin 1/20, Loestrin Fe 1/20, Microgestin Fe 1/20, Minastrin 24 Fe

THERAPEUTIC CLASS:
Contraceptive (monophasic)

GENERAL USES:
Contraception

DOSAGE FORMS:
Tablets: 20 mcg/1 mg

ETHINYL ESTRADIOL/ NORETHINDRONE

ETH in il es tra DYE ole/nor eth IN drone

TRADE NAME(S):
Jenest-28, Nelova 10/11, Ortho-Novum 10/11, Necon 10/11

THERAPEUTIC CLASS:
Contraceptive (biphasic)

General Uses:
Contraception

Dosage Forms:
Tablets: Phase 1:
35 mcg/0.5 mg; Phase 2:
35 mcg/1 mg

ETHINYL ESTRADIOL/ NORETHINDRONE

ETH in il es tra DYE ole/nor
eth IN drone

Trade Name(s):
Tri-Norinyl

Therapeutic Class:
Contraceptive (triphasic)

General Uses:
Contraception

Dosage Forms:
Tablets: Phase 1:
35 mcg/0.5 mg; Phase 2:
35 mcg/1 mg; Phase 3:
35 mcg/0.5 mg

ETHINYL ESTRADIOL/ NORETHINDRONE

ETH in il es tra DYE ole/nor
eth IN drone

Trade Name(s):
Ortho-Novum 7/7/7,
Necon 7/7/7

Therapeutic Class:
Contraceptive (triphasic)

General Uses:
Contraception

Dosage Forms:
Tablets: Phase 1:
35 mcg/0.5 mg; Phase 2:

35 mcg/0.75 mg; Phase
3: 35 mcg/1 mg

ETHINYL ESTRADIOL/ NORETHINDRONE

ETH in il es tra DYE ole/nor
eth IN drone

Trade Name(s):
Estrostep, Estrostep Fe

Therapeutic Class:
Contraceptive (triphasic)

General Uses:
Contraception

Dosage Forms:
Tablets: Phase 1:
20 mcg/1 mg; Phase 2:
30 mcg/1 mg; Phase 3:
35 mcg/1 mg

ETHINYL ESTRADIOL/ NORETHINDRONE

ETH in il es tra DYE ole/nor
eth IN drone

Trade Name(s):
Lo Minastrin Fe

Therapeutic Class:
Contraceptive

General Uses:
Contraception

Dosage Forms:
Tablets: Phase 1:
10 mcg/1 mg; Phase 2:
10 mcg/0 mg

ETHINYL ESTRADIOL/ NORGESTIMATE
ETH in il es tra DYE ole/nor JES ti mate

TRADE NAME(S):
Ortho-Cyclen, Sprintec

THERAPEUTIC CLASS:
Contraceptive (monophasic)

GENERAL USES:
Contraception

DOSAGE FORMS:
Tablets: 35 mcg/0.25 mg

ETHINYL ESTRADIOL/ NORGESTIMATE
ETH in il es tra DYE ole/nor JES ti mate

TRADE NAME(S):
Ortho-Cyclen, Ortho-Tri-Cyclen, Sprintec

THERAPEUTIC CLASS:
Contraceptive (triphasic)

GENERAL USES:
Contraception

DOSAGE FORMS:
Tablets: Phase 1: 35 mcg/0.18 mg; Phase 2: 35 mcg/0.215 mg; Phase 3: 35 mcg/0.25 mg

ETHINYL ESTRADIOL/ NORGESTREL
ETH in il es tra DYE ole/nor JES trel

TRADE NAME(S):
Ovral, Ogestrel

THERAPEUTIC CLASS:
Contraceptive (monophasic)

GENERAL USES:
Contraception

DOSAGE FORMS:
Tablets: 50 mcg/0.5 mg

ETHINYL ESTRADIOL/ NORGESTREL
ETH in il es tra DYE ole/nor JES trel

TRADE NAME(S):
Cryselle, Lo/Ovral, Low-Ogestrel

THERAPEUTIC CLASS:
Contraceptive (monophasic)

GENERAL USES:
Contraception

DOSAGE FORMS:
Tablets: 30 mcg/0.3 mg

ETHIONAMIDE
e thye on AM ide

TRADE NAME(S):
Trecator-SC

THERAPEUTIC CLASS:
Antituberculosis agent

GENERAL USES:
Tuberculosis

DOSAGE FORMS:
Tablets: 250 mg

ETHOSUXIMIDE
eth oh SUKS i mide

TRADE NAME(S):
Zarontin

THERAPEUTIC CLASS:
Anticonvulsant
GENERAL USES:
Seizures
DOSAGE FORMS:
Capsules: 250 mg; Syrup: 250 mg/5 mL

ETIDRONATE
e ti DROE nate
TRADE NAME(S):
Didronel
THERAPEUTIC CLASS:
Bisphosphonate
GENERAL USES:
Paget's disease, hypercalcemia (cancer related)
DOSAGE FORMS:
Tablets: 200 mg, 400 mg

ETODOLAC
ee toe DOE lak
TRADE NAME(S):
Lodine, Lodine XL
THERAPEUTIC CLASS:
Anti-inflammatory/ analgesic
GENERAL USES:
Osteoarthritis, rheumatoid arthritis, ankylosing spondylitis, pain
DOSAGE FORMS:
Tablets: 400 mg, 500 mg; Extended-release tablets: 400 mg, 500 mg, 600 mg; Capsules: 200 mg, 300 mg

ETONOGESTREL
et oh noe JES trel
TRADE NAME(S):
Implanon
THERAPEUTIC CLASS:
Contraceptive
GENERAL USES:
Contraception
DOSAGE FORMS:
Implant: 68 mg

ETRAVIRINE
e tra VEER een
TRADE NAME(S):
Intelence
THERAPEUTIC CLASS:
Antiviral
GENERAL USES:
HIV infection
DOSAGE FORMS:
Tablets: 25 mg, 100 mg, 200 mg

ETRETINATE
ee TRET ih nate
TRADE NAME(S):
Tegison
THERAPEUTIC CLASS:
Retinoid
GENERAL USES:
Psoriasis
DOSAGE FORMS:
Capsules: 10 mg, 25 mg

EVEROLIMUS
E ver OH li mus
TRADE NAME(S):
Afinitor, Disperz, Zortress

THERAPEUTIC CLASS:
Antineoplastic

GENERAL USES:
Various cancers, prevent organ rejection in kidney and liver transplants

DOSAGE FORMS:
Tablets: 0.25 mg, 0.5 mg, 0.75 mg, 2.5 mg, 5 mg, 10 mg; Tablets for suspension: 2 mg, 3 mg, 5 mg

EXEMESTANE
ex e MES tane

TRADE NAME(S):
Aromasin

THERAPEUTIC CLASS:
Antineoplastic

GENERAL USES:
Breast cancer

DOSAGE FORMS:
Tablets: 25 mg

EXENATIDE
ex EN a tide

TRADE NAME(S):
Byetta, Bydureon

THERAPEUTIC CLASS:
Antidiabetic

GENERAL USES:
Diabetes (type 2)

DOSAGE FORMS:
Injection: 250 mcg/mL, 2 mg

EXENATIDE (SYNTHETIC)
ex EN a tide

TRADE NAME(S):
Bydureon

THERAPEUTIC CLASS:
Antidiabetic

GENERAL USES:
Diabetes (type 2)

DOSAGE FORMS:
Injection (extended release): 2 mg

EZETIMIBE
ez ET i mibe

TRADE NAME(S):
Zetia

THERAPEUTIC CLASS:
Antilipemic

GENERAL USES:
Hyperlipidemia

DOSAGE FORMS:
Tablets: 10 mg

EZETIMIBE/ ATORVASTATIN
ez ET i mibe/a TORE va sta tin

TRADE NAME(S):
Liptruzet

THERAPEUTIC CLASS:
Antilipemic

GENERAL USES:
Hypercholesterolemia

DOSAGE FORMS:
Tablets: 10 mg/10 mg, 10 mg/20 mg, 10 mg/40 mg, 10 mg/80 mg

**EZETIMIBE/
SIMVASTATIN**
ez ET i mibe/SIM va stat in
TRADE NAME(S):
Vytorin
THERAPEUTIC CLASS:
Antilipemic
GENERAL USES:
Hypercholesterolemia
DOSAGE FORMS:
Tablets: 10 mg/10 mg,
10 mg/20 mg, 10 mg/
40 mg, 10 mg/80 mg

EZOGABINE
e ZOG a been
TRADE NAME(S):
Potiga
THERAPEUTIC CLASS:
Anticonvulsant
GENERAL USES:
Seizures
DOSAGE FORMS:
Tablets: 50 mg, 200 mg,
300 mg, 400 mg

**FACTOR XIII
CONCENTRATE
(HUMAN)**
FAK tor
TRADE NAME(S):
Corifact
THERAPEUTIC CLASS:
Hematological agent
GENERAL USES:
Factor XIII deficiency

DOSAGE FORMS:
Injection: 1000 to 1600
units

FAMCICLOVIR
fam SYE kloe veer
TRADE NAME(S):
Famvir
THERAPEUTIC CLASS:
Antiviral
GENERAL USES:
Herpes, shingles
DOSAGE FORMS:
Tablets: 125 mg, 250 mg,
500 mg

FAMOTIDINE
fa MOE ti deen
TRADE NAME(S):
Pepcid, Pepcid AC,
Pepcid RPD
THERAPEUTIC CLASS:
Gastric acid secretion
inhibitor
GENERAL USES:
GERD, GI ulcers
DOSAGE FORMS:
Tablets: 10 mg, 20 mg,
40 mg; Chewable tablets:
10 mg; Suspension:
40 mg/5 mL; Injection:
20 mg, 40 mg

FEBUXOSTAT
feb UX oh stat
TRADE NAME(S):
Uloric

THERAPEUTIC CLASS:
Gout agent
GENERAL USES:
Gout
DOSAGE FORMS:
Tablets: 40 mg, 80 mg

FELODIPINE
fe LOE di peen
TRADE NAME(S):
Plendil
THERAPEUTIC CLASS:
Antihypertensive
GENERAL USES:
Hypertension
DOSAGE FORMS:
Extended-release tablets:
2.5 mg, 5 mg, 10 mg

FENOFIBRATE
fen oh FYE brate
TRADE NAME(S):
TriCor, Antara, Triglide,
Lipofen
THERAPEUTIC CLASS:
Antilipemic
GENERAL USES:
Hyperlipidemia
DOSAGE FORMS:
Capsules: 43 mg, 50 mg,
67 mg, 87 mg, 130 mg,
134 mg, 150 mg, 200 mg;
Tablets: 48 mg, 50 mg,
145 mg

FENOFIBRIC ACID
FEN oh FYE bric
TRADE NAME(S):
Fibricor, Trilipix

THERAPEUTIC CLASS:
Antilipemic
GENERAL USES:
Hyperlipidemia
DOSAGE FORMS:
Delayed-release capsules:
45 mg, 135 mg; Tablets:
35 mg, 105 mg

FENOPROFEN
fen oh PROE fen
TRADE NAME(S):
Nalfon
THERAPEUTIC CLASS:
Anti-inflammatory/
analgesic
GENERAL USES:
Osteoarthritis, rheumatoid
arthritis, pain
DOSAGE FORMS:
Capsules: 200 mg,
300 mg; Tablets: 600 mg

FENTANYL (BUCCAL)
FEN ta nil
TRADE NAME(S):
Fentora, Onsolis
THERAPEUTIC CLASS:
Analgesic (narcotic)
GENERAL USES:
Pain
DOSAGE FORMS:
Buccal film: 200 mcg,
400 mcg, 600 mcg,
800 mcg, 1200 mcg;
Buccal tablets: 100 mcg,
200 mcg, 400 mcg,
600 mcg, 800 mcg

FENTANYL (INJECTION)
FEN ta nil
TRADE NAME(S):
  Sublimaze
THERAPEUTIC CLASS:
  Analgesic (narcotic)
GENERAL USES:
  Premedicant for
  anesthesia
DOSAGE FORMS:
  Injection: 0.1 mg,
  0.25 mg, 0.5 mg, 1 mg,
  1.5 mg, 2.5 mg

FENTANYL (NASAL)
FEN ta nil
TRADE NAME(S):
  Lazanda
THERAPEUTIC CLASS:
  Analgesic (narcotic)
GENERAL USES:
  Breakthrough cancer pain
DOSAGE FORMS:
  Nasal spray: 100 mcg,
  400 mcg

FENTANYL (ORAL)
FEN ta nil
TRADE NAME(S):
  Actiq, Oralet
THERAPEUTIC CLASS:
  Analgesic (narcotic)
GENERAL USES:
  Pain, pre-op medication
DOSAGE FORMS:
  Lozenge: 200 mcg,
  300 mcg, 400 mcg;

Lozenge/stick: 200 mcg,
400 mcg, 600 mcg,
800 mcg, 1200 mcg,
1600 mcg

**FENTANYL
(SUBLINGUAL)**
FEN ta nil
TRADE NAME(S):
  Abstral, Subsys
THERAPEUTIC CLASS:
  Analgesic (narcotic)
GENERAL USES:
  Breakthrough cancer pain
DOSAGE FORMS:
  Sublingual spray: 100 mcg,
  200 mcg, 400 mcg,
  600 mcg, 800 mcg;
  Sublingual tablets:
  100 mcg, 200 mcg,
  300 mcg, 400 mcg,
  600 mcg, 800 mcg

**FENTANYL
(TRANSDERMAL)**
FEN ta nil
TRADE NAME(S):
  Duragesic
THERAPEUTIC CLASS:
  Analgesic (narcotic)
GENERAL USES:
  Pain
DOSAGE FORMS:
  Transdermal patch (mcg/
  hr): 25, 50, 75, 100

FERRIC CARBOXYMALTOSE
FER ik kar BOKS ee MAWL tose

TRADE NAME(S):
Injectafer

THERAPEUTIC CLASS:
Iron product

GENERAL USES:
Iron deficiency anemia

DOSAGE FORMS:
Injection: 750 mg

FERRIC CITRATE
FER ik

TRADE NAME(S):
Ferric citrate

THERAPEUTIC CLASS:
Phosphate-binding agent

GENERAL CLASS:
High phosphorous levels in kidney disease

DOSAGE FORMS:
Tablets: 1 g

FERUMOXYTOL
FER yoo MOKS i tol

TRADE NAME(S):
Feraheme

THERAPEUTIC CLASS:
Hematological agent

GENERAL USES:
Iron deficiency anemia

DOSAGE FORMS:
Injection: 510 mg

FESOTERODINE FUMARATE
FES oh TER oh deen fyoo MAR ate

TRADE NAME(S):
Toviaz

THERAPEUTIC CLASS:
Anticholinergic

GENERAL USES:
Overactive bladder

DOSAGE FORMS:
Extended-release tablets: 4 mg, 8 mg

FEXOFENADINE
feks oh FEN a deen

TRADE NAME(S):
Allegra

THERAPEUTIC CLASS:
Antihistamine

GENERAL USES:
Allergic rhinitis, chronic hives

DOSAGE FORMS:
Tablets: 30 mg, 60 mg, 180 mg; Oral suspension: 6 mg/mL

FEXOFENADINE/ PSEUDOEPHEDRINE
feks oh FEN a deen/soo doe e FED rin

TRADE NAME(S):
Allegra-D 12 Hour, Allegra-D 24 Hour

THERAPEUTIC CLASS:
Antihistamine/ decongestant

GENERAL USES:
Allergic rhinitis
DOSAGE FORMS:
Extended-release tablets:
60 mg/120 mg,
180 mg/240 mg

FIDAXOMICIN
fye DAX oh MYE sin
TRADE NAME(S):
Dificid
THERAPEUTIC CLASS:
Anti-infective
GENERAL USES:
Clostridium difficile-
related diarrhea
DOSAGE FORMS:
Tablets: 200 mg

FINASTERIDE
fi NAS teer ide
TRADE NAME(S):
Propecia, Proscar
THERAPEUTIC CLASS:
Antiandrogen
GENERAL USES:
Male-pattern baldness,
BPH
DOSAGE FORMS:
Tablets: 1 mg, 5 mg

FINGOLIMOD
fin GOLE i mod
TRADE NAME(S):
Gilenya
THERAPEUTIC CLASS:
Multiple sclerosis agent
GENERAL USES:
Multiple sclerosis

DOSAGE FORMS:
Capsules: 0.5 mg

FLECAINIDE
fle KAY nide
TRADE NAME(S):
Tambocor
THERAPEUTIC CLASS:
Antiarrhythmic
GENERAL USES:
Atrial fibrillation,
tachycardia, arrhythmias
DOSAGE FORMS:
Tablets: 50 mg, 100 mg,
150 mg

FLORBETABEN F-18
flor BAY ta ben
TRADE NAME(S):
Neuraceq
THERAPEUTIC CLASS:
Radioactive agent
GENERAL USES:
Brain imaging
DOSAGE FORMS:
Injection: 30 mL

FLORBETAPIR F 18
flor BAY ta peer
TRADE NAME(S):
Amyvid
THERAPEUTIC CLASS:
Radioactive agent
GENERAL USES:
Brain imaging
DOSAGE FORMS:
Injection: 10 mL, 30 mL,
50 mL

FLUCONAZOLE
floo KOE na zole
TRADE NAME(S):
Diflucan, Diflucan IV
THERAPEUTIC CLASS:
Antifungal
GENERAL USES:
Fungal infections
DOSAGE FORMS:
Tablets: 50 mg, 100 mg,
150 mg, 200 mg;
Suspension: 10 mg/mL,
40 mg/mL; Injection:
200 mg, 400 mg

FLUCYTOSINE
floo SYE toe seen
TRADE NAME(S):
Ancobon
THERAPEUTIC CLASS:
Antifungal
GENERAL USES:
Fungal infections
DOSAGE FORMS:
Capsules: 250 mg, 500 mg

FLUNISOLIDE (INHALED)
floo NISS oh lide
TRADE NAME(S):
AeroBid, Aerospan
THERAPEUTIC CLASS:
Corticosteroid (inhaler)
GENERAL USES:
Asthma (chronic)
DOSAGE FORMS:
Inhaler: 250 mcg/
inhalation, 80 mg/
inhalation

FLUNISOLIDE (NASAL)
floo NISS oh lide
TRADE NAME(S):
Nasalide, Nasarel
THERAPEUTIC CLASS:
Corticosteroid (nasal)
GENERAL USES:
Allergies
DOSAGE FORMS:
Nasal spray: 0.025%

FLUOCINOLONE
floo oh SIN oh lone
TRADE NAME(S):
Synalar, Fluonid,
Flurosyn
THERAPEUTIC CLASS:
Corticosteroid (topical)
GENERAL USES:
Various skin conditions
DOSAGE FORMS:
Ointment: 0.025%;
Cream: 0.01%, 0.025%,
0.2%; Solution: 0.01%

FLUOCINOLONE ACETONIDE (IMPLANT)
floo oh SIN oh lone ah SEE
toe nide
TRADE NAME(S):
Iluvien, Retisert
THERAPEUTIC CLASS:
Ocular agent
GENERAL USES:
Noninfectious
uveitis

DOSAGE FORMS:
Intravitreal implant: 0.19
mg, 0.59 mg

FLUOCINONIDE
floo oh SIN oh nide
TRADE NAME(S):
Lidex, Fluonex, Vanos
THERAPEUTIC CLASS:
Corticosteroid (topical)
GENERAL USES:
Various skin conditions
DOSAGE FORMS:
Cream, Ointment,
Solution, and Gel: 0.05%;
Cream: 0.1%

FLUOROMETHOLONE
flure oh METH oh lone
TRADE NAME(S):
Fluor-Op, FML, Flarex
THERAPEUTIC CLASS:
Ocular agent (steroid)
GENERAL USES:
Ocular inflammation
DOSAGE FORMS:
Ophthalmic
suspension: 0.1%, 0.25%;
Ophthalmic ointment:
0.1%

**FLUOROURACIL
(INJECTION)**
flure oh YOOR a sil
TRADE NAME(S):
Adrucil, 5-FU
THERAPEUTIC CLASS:
Antineoplastic

GENERAL USES:
Cancers of the colon,
rectum, breast,
stomach, and pancreas
DOSAGE FORMS:
Injection: 500 mg, 1 g,
2.5 g, 5 g

**FLUOROURACIL
(TOPICAL)**
flure oh YOOR a sil
TRADE NAME(S):
Efudex, Fluoroplex
THERAPEUTIC CLASS:
Antineoplastic
GENERAL USES:
Skin disorders
DOSAGE FORMS:
Cream: 1%, 5%;
Solution: 1%, 2%, 5%

FLUOXETINE
floo OKS e teen
TRADE NAME(S):
Prozac, Prozac Weekly,
Sarafem
THERAPEUTIC CLASS:
Antidepressant
GENERAL USES:
Depression, bulimia,
OCD, PMDD
DOSAGE FORMS:
Tablets: 10 mg, 15 mg,
20 mg, 60 mg; Capsules:
10 mg, 20 mg, 40 mg,
60 mg; Solution:
20 mg/5 mL; Delayed-
release capsules: 90 mg

FLUPHENAZINE
floo FEN a zeen
TRADE NAME(S):
Prolixin, Permitil
THERAPEUTIC CLASS:
Antipsychotic
GENERAL USES:
Psychotic disorders
DOSAGE FORMS:
Tablets: 1 mg,
2.5 mg, 5 mg, 10 mg;
Elixir: 2.5 mg/5 mL;
Concentrated solution:
5 mg/mL

FLURAZEPAM
flure AZ e pam
TRADE NAME(S):
Dalmane
THERAPEUTIC CLASS:
Sedative/hypnotic
GENERAL USES:
Insomnia
DOSAGE FORMS:
Capsules: 15 mg, 30 mg

**FLURBIPROFEN
(OCULAR)**
flur BI proe fen
TRADE NAME(S):
Ocufen
THERAPEUTIC CLASS:
Ocular agent
GENERAL USES:
Maintain pupil dilation
during surgery

DOSAGE FORMS:
Ophthalmic solution:
0.03%

FLURBIPROFEN (ORAL)
flur BI proe fen
TRADE NAME(S):
Ansaid
THERAPEUTIC CLASS:
Anti-inflammatory/
analgesic
GENERAL USES:
Osteoarthritis, rheumatoid
arthritis
DOSAGE FORMS:
Tablets: 50 mg, 100 mg

FLUTAMIDE
FLOO ta mide
TRADE NAME(S):
Eulexin
THERAPEUTIC CLASS:
Antiandrogen/
antineoplastic
GENERAL USES:
Prostate cancer
DOSAGE FORMS:
Capsules: 125 mg

FLUTEMETAMOL F-18
floo te MET a mol
TRADE NAME(S):
Vizamyl
THERAPEUTIC CLASS:
Radioactive agent
GENERAL USES:
Brain imaging

DOSAGE FORMS:
Injection: 10 mL, 30 mL

FLUTICASONE (INHALED)
floo TIK a sone
TRADE NAME(S):
Flovent HFA, Flovent Rotadisk, Flovent Diskus, Arnuity Ellipta
THERAPEUTIC CLASS:
Corticosteroid (inhaler)
GENERAL USES:
Asthma (chronic)
DOSAGE FORMS:
Aerosol: 44 mcg/actuation, 110 mcg/actuation, 220 mcg/actuation; Inhaler: 50 mcg/actuation, 100 mcg/actuation, 200 mg/actuation, 250 mcg/actuation

FLUTICASONE FUROATE/VILANTEROL TRIFENATATE
floo TIK a sone/vye LAN ter ol
TRADE NAME(S):
BREO Ellipta
THERAPEUTIC CLASS:
Corticosteroid/bronchodilator
GENERAL USES:
COPD

DOSAGE FORMS:
Inhalation: 100 mcg/25 mcg/double blister strip

FLUTICASONE (NASAL)
floo TIK a sone
TRADE NAME(S):
Flonase, Veramyst
THERAPEUTIC CLASS:
Corticosteroid (nasal)
GENERAL USES:
Allergies
DOSAGE FORMS:
Nasal spray: 50 mcg/spray, 27.5 mcg/spray

FLUTICASONE PROPIONATE (TOPICAL)
floo TIK a sone
TRADE NAME(S):
Cutivate
THERAPEUTIC CLASS:
Corticosteroid (topical)
GENERAL USES:
Various skin conditions
DOSAGE FORMS:
Cream: 0.05%; Ointment: 0.005%

FLUTICASONE/ SALMETEROL
floo TIK a sone/sal ME te role
TRADE NAME(S):
Advair Diskus
THERAPEUTIC CLASS:
Corticosteroid/bronchodilator

GENERAL USES:
  Asthma (chronic), COPD
DOSAGE FORMS:
  Inhalation: 0.1 mg/
  0.05 mg/inhalation,
  0.25 mg/0.05 mg/
  inhalation, 0.5 mg/
  0.05 mg/inhalation

FLUVASTATIN
FLOO va sta tin
TRADE NAME(S):
  Lescol, Lescol XL
THERAPEUTIC CLASS:
  Antilipemic
GENERAL USES:
  Hyperlipidemia,
  secondary prevention of
  CHD
DOSAGE FORMS:
  Capsules: 20 mg, 40 mg;
  Extended-release tablets:
  80 mg

FLUVOXAMINE
floo VOKS a meen
TRADE NAME(S):
  Luvox, Luvox CR
THERAPEUTIC CLASS:
  Antidepressant
GENERAL USES:
  OCD
DOSAGE FORMS:
  Tablets: 25 mg, 50 mg,
  100 mg; Extended-release
  capsules: 100 mg, 150 mg

FOLIC ACID/ CYANOCOBALAMIN/ PYRIDOXINE
FOE lik AS id/sye an oh koe
BAL a min/peer i DOKS een
TRADE NAME(S):
  Foltx
THERAPEUTIC CLASS:
  Vitamin
GENERAL USES:
  Nutritional
  supplementation
DOSAGE FORMS:
  Tablets: 2.5 mg/1 mg/
  25 mg

FONDAPARINUX SODIUM
fon da PARE i nuks
TRADE NAME(S):
  Arixtra
THERAPEUTIC CLASS:
  Anticoagulant (LMWH)
GENERAL USES:
  Prevention of blood clots
DOSAGE FORMS:
  Injection: 2.5 mg

FORMOTEROL
for MOE te rol
TRADE NAME(S):
  Foradil
THERAPEUTIC CLASS:
  Bronchodilator
GENERAL USES:
  Asthma (chronic)

Dosage Forms:
  Inhalation: 12 mcg/
  inhalation

FORMOTEROL FUMARATE
for MOE te rol fyoo MAR ate
Trade Name(s):
  Perforomist
Therapeutic Class:
  Bronchodilator
General Uses:
  COPD
Dosage Forms:
  Inhalation solution:
  20 mcg/2 mL

FORMOTEROL FUMARATE/ MOMETASONE (INHALATION)
for MOE ter ol fyoo MAR ate/
moe MET a sone
Trade Name(s):
  Dulera
Therapeutic Class:
  Bronchodilator/
  corticosteroid
General Uses:
  Asthma
Dosage Forms:
  Inhalation solution (oral):
  100 mcg/5 mcg,
  200 mcg/5 mcg

FOSAMPRENAVIR
FOS am pren a veer
Trade Name(s):
  Lexiva
Therapeutic Class:
  Antiviral
General Uses:
  HIV infection
Dosage Forms:
  Tablets: 700 mg; Oral
  suspension: 50 mg/mL

FOSAPREPITANT DIMEGLUMINE
FOS ap RE pi tant dye MEG
loo meen
Trade Name(s):
  Emend
Therapeutic Class:
  Antiemetic
General Uses:
  Chemotherapy-induced
  nausea/vomiting
Dosage Forms:
  Injection: 115 mg

FOSCARNET
fos KAR net
Trade Name(s):
  Foscavir
Therapeutic Class:
  Antiviral
General Uses:
  CMV retinitis, herpes
  simplex virus
  infections
Dosage Forms:
  Injection: 12 g

FOSINOPRIL
foe SIN oh pril
TRADE NAME(S):
Monopril
THERAPEUTIC CLASS:
Antihypertensive, cardiac
agent
GENERAL USES:
Hypertension, heart failure
DOSAGE FORMS:
Tablets: 10 mg, 20 mg,
40 mg

FOSPHENYTOIN
FOS fen i toyn
TRADE NAME(S):
Cerebyx
THERAPEUTIC CLASS:
Anticonvulsant
GENERAL USES:
Seizures
DOSAGE FORMS:
Injection: 150 mg, 750 mg

**FOSPROPOFOL
DISODIUM**
fos proe POE fol
TRADE NAME(S):
Lusedra
THERAPEUTIC CLASS:
Sedative
GENERAL USES:
Sedation with anesthesia
in surgery
DOSAGE FORMS:
Injection: 1050 mg

FROVATRIPTAN
froe va TRIP tan
TRADE NAME(S):
Frova
THERAPEUTIC CLASS:
Antimigraine agent
GENERAL USES:
Acute treatment of
migraine
DOSAGE FORMS:
Tablets: 2.5 mg

FULVESTRANT
fool VES trant
TRADE NAME(S):
Faslodex
THERAPEUTIC CLASS:
Antineoplastic
GENERAL USES:
Breast cancer
DOSAGE FORMS:
Injection: 250 mg

FUROSEMIDE
fyoor OH se mide
TRADE NAME(S):
Lasix
THERAPEUTIC CLASS:
Diuretic
GENERAL USES:
CHF- and pulmonary-
related edema,
hypertension
DOSAGE FORMS:
Tablets: 20 mg, 40 mg,
80 mg; Solution:

10 mg/mL, 40 mg/5 mL;
Injection: 20 mg, 40 mg,
100 mg

GABAPENTIN
GAB a PEN tin
TRADE NAME(S):
Gralise, Neurontin
THERAPEUTIC CLASS:
Anticonvulsant
GENERAL USES:
Seizures, postherpetic
neuralgia
DOSAGE FORMS:
Capsules: 100 mg,
300 mg, 400 mg; Tablets:
100 mg, 300 mg, 400 mg,
600 mg, 800 mg;
Solution: 250 mg/5 mL

GABAPENTIN ENACARBIL
GAB a PEN tin EN a KAR bil
TRADE NAME(S):
Horizant
THERAPEUTIC CLASS:
Analgesic
GENERAL USES:
Restless leg syndrome,
shingles pain
DOSAGE FORMS:
Extended-release tablets:
300 mg, 600 mg

GADOBENATE DIMEGLUMINE
gad oh BEN ate
dye MEG loo meen
TRADE NAME(S):
Multihance
THERAPEUTIC CLASS:
Radiopaque agent
GENERAL USES:
Enhancement of MRI
DOSAGE FORMS:
Injection: 2.645 g,
5.290 g, 7.935 g, 10.58 g,
26.45 g, 52.9 g

GADOBUTROL
GAD oh BUE trol
TRADE NAME(S):
Gadavist
THERAPEUTIC CLASS:
Radiopaque agent
GENERAL USES:
Magnetic resonance
imaging of CNS
DOSAGE FORMS:
Injection: 1 mmol/mL

GADOFOSVESET TRISODIUM
GAD oh FOS ve set
TRADE NAME(S):
Ablavar
THERAPEUTIC CLASS:
Radiopaque agent
GENERAL USES:
Magnetic resonance
angiography of peripheral

vascular disease

DOSAGE FORMS:
Injection: 2440 mg,
3660 mg

GADOTERATE MEGLUMINE
gad oh TER ate MEG loo
meen

TRADE NAME(S):
Dotarem

THERAPEUTIC CLASS:
Radiopaque agent

GENERAL USES:
Enhancement of MRI

DOSAGE FORMS:
Injection: 3.769 g, 5.6535
g, 7.538 g, 37.69 g

GADOXETATE DISODIUM
ga DOKS e tate

TRADE NAME(S):
Eovist

THERAPEUTIC CLASS:
Radiopaque agent

GENERAL USES:
MRI of liver

DOSAGE FORMS:
Injection: 10 mL

GALANTAMINE
ga LAN ta meen

TRADE NAME(S):
Razadyne ER, Razadyne

THERAPEUTIC CLASS:
Alzheimer's agent

GENERAL USES:
Mild to moderate
dementia of Alzheimer's

DOSAGE FORMS:
Tablets: 4 mg, 8 mg,
12 mg; Solution: 4 mg/
mL; Extended-release
capsules: 8 mg, 16 mg,
24 mg

GALSULFASE
gal SUL fase

TRADE NAME(S):
Naglazyme

THERAPEUTIC CLASS:
Enzyme

GENERAL USES:
Mucopolysaccharidosis VI

DOSAGE FORMS:
Injection: 5 mg

GANCICLOVIR
gan SYE kloe veer

TRADE NAME(S):
Cytovene, Zirgan

THERAPEUTIC CLASS:
Antiviral

GENERAL USES:
CMV retinitis and
infection

DOSAGE FORMS:
Gel: 0.15%; Injection:
500 mg

GATIFLOXACIN (OCULAR)
ga ti FLOKS a sin

TRADE NAME(S):
Zymar, Zymaxid
THERAPEUTIC CLASS:
Ocular agent (anti-infective)
GENERAL USES:
Ocular infections
DOSAGE FORMS:
Ophthalmic solution: 0.3%, 0.5%

GEFITINIB
ge FI tye nib
TRADE NAME(S):
Iressa
THERAPEUTIC CLASS:
Antineoplastic
GENERAL USES:
Non-small-cell lung cancer
DOSAGE FORMS:
Tablets: 250 mg

GEMFIBROZIL
jem FI broe zil
TRADE NAME(S):
Lopid
THERAPEUTIC CLASS:
Antilipemic
GENERAL USES:
Hyperlipidemia
DOSAGE FORMS:
Tablets: 600 mg

GEMIFLOXACIN
je mi FLOKS a sin
TRADE NAME(S):
Factive

THERAPEUTIC CLASS:
Anti-infective
GENERAL USES:
Bacterial infections
DOSAGE FORMS:
Tablets: 320 mg

GENTAMICIN
jen ta MYE sin
TRADE NAME(S):
Garamycin, Genoptic, Gentak
THERAPEUTIC CLASS:
Ocular agent (anti-infective)
GENERAL USES:
Ocular infections
DOSAGE FORMS:
Ophthalmic ointment: 3 mg/g; Ophthalmic solution: 3 mg/mL

GENTAMICIN (INJECTION)
jen ta MYE sin
TRADE NAME(S):
Garamycin
THERAPEUTIC CLASS:
Anti-infective
GENERAL USES:
Bacterial infections
DOSAGE FORMS:
Injection: 20 mg, 60 mg, 80 mg, 800 mg

GLATIRAMER ACETATE
gla TIR a mer AS e tate
TRADE NAME(S):
Copaxone

THERAPEUTIC CLASS:
Miscellaneous
GENERAL USES:
Multiple sclerosis
DOSAGE FORMS:
Injection: 20 mg, 40 mg

GLIMEPIRIDE
GLYE me pye ride
TRADE NAME(S):
Amaryl
THERAPEUTIC CLASS:
Antidiabetic
GENERAL USES:
Diabetes (type 2)
DOSAGE FORMS:
Tablets: 1 mg, 2 mg, 4 mg

GLIPIZIDE
GLIP i zide
TRADE NAME(S):
Glipizide XL, Glucotrol,
Glucotrol XL
THERAPEUTIC CLASS:
Antidiabetic
GENERAL USES:
Diabetes (type 2)
DOSAGE FORMS:
Tablets: 5 mg, 10 mg;
Extended-release tablets:
2.5 mg, 5 mg, 10 mg

GLUCARPIDASE
gloo KAR pi dayz
TRADE NAME(S):
Voraxaze
THERAPEUTIC CLASS:
Enzyme

GENERAL USES:
Toxic methotrexate levels
DOSAGE FORMS:
Injection: 1000 units

GLYBURIDE
GLYE byoor ide
TRADE NAME(S):
Diabeta, Micronase,
Glynase
THERAPEUTIC CLASS:
Antidiabetic
GENERAL USES:
Diabetes (type 2)
DOSAGE FORMS:
Tablets: 1.25 mg, 2.5 mg,
5 mg; Micronized tablets:
1.5 mg, 3 mg, 4.5 mg,
6 mg

GLYBURIDE/ METFORMIN
GLYE byoor ide/met FOR
min
TRADE NAME(S):
Glucovance
THERAPEUTIC CLASS:
Antidiabetic
GENERAL USES:
Diabetes (type 2)
DOSAGE FORMS:
Tablets: 1.25 mg/250 mg,
2.5 mg/500 mg, 5 mg/
500 mg

GLYCEROL PHENYLBUTYRATE
GLIS er ol FEN il BYOO ti rate

TRADE NAME(S):
Ravicti

THERAPEUTIC CLASS:
Hyperammonemia agent

GENERAL USES:
Urea cycle disorders

DOSAGE FORMS:
Oral liquid: 1.1 g/mL

GLYCOPYRROLATE
glye koe PYE roe late

TRADE NAME(S):
Cuvposa

THERAPEUTIC CLASS:
Anticholinergic

GENERAL USES:
Severe, chronic drooling

DOSAGE FORMS:
Oral solution: 1 mg/5 mL

GOLIMUMAB
goe LIM yoo mab

TRADE NAME(S):
Simponi, Simponi Aria

THERAPEUTIC CLASS:
Monoclonal antibody

GENERAL USES:
Rheumatoid arthritis, psoriatic arthritis, ankylosing spondylitis, ulcerative colitis

DOSAGE FORMS:
Injection: 50 mg, 100 mg

GRANISETRON
gra NIS e tron

TRADE NAME(S):
Kytril

THERAPEUTIC CLASS:
Antiemetic

GENERAL USES:
Postoperative chemotherapy nausea/vomiting

DOSAGE FORMS:
Tablets: 1 mg; Injection: 1 mg, 4 mg; Oral solution: 2 mg/10 mL

GRANISETRON (TRANSDERMAL)
gra NIS e tron

TRADE NAME(S):
Sancuso

THERAPEUTIC CLASS:
Antiemetic

GENERAL USES:
Chemotherapy nausea/vomiting

DOSAGE FORMS:
Patch: 3.1 mg/24 hr

GRISEOFULVIN MICROSIZE
gri see oh FUL vin

TRADE NAME(S):
Fulvicin, Grifulvin

THERAPEUTIC CLASS:
Antifungal

GENERAL USES:
Fungal infections

DOSAGE FORMS:
Tablets: 250 mg,
500 mg;
Capsules: 125 mg,
250 mg; Suspension:
125 mg/5 mL

GRISEOFULVIN ULTRAMICROSIZE
gri see oh FUL vin
TRADE NAME(S):
Fulvicin P/G, Grisactin,
Gris-PEG
THERAPEUTIC CLASS:
Antifungal
GENERAL USES:
Fungal infections
DOSAGE FORMS:
Tablets: 125 mg, 165 mg,
250 mg, 330 mg

GUAIFENESIN/ PSEUDOEPHEDRINE
gwye FEN e sin/soo doe e
FED rin
TRADE NAME(S):
Guaifenex PSE
THERAPEUTIC CLASS:
Mucolytic/decongestant
GENERAL USES:
Cough and colds
DOSAGE FORMS:
Sustained-release tablets:
600 mg/60 mg,
600 mg/120 mg,
1200 mg/60 mg,
1200 mg/120 mg

GUANABENZ
GWAHN a benz
TRADE NAME(S):
Wytensin
THERAPEUTIC CLASS:
Antihypertensive
GENERAL USES:
Hypertension
DOSAGE FORMS:
Tablets: 4 mg, 8 mg

GUANADREL
GWAHN a drel
TRADE NAME(S):
Hylorel
THERAPEUTIC CLASS:
Antihypertensive
GENERAL USES:
Hypertension
DOSAGE FORMS:
Tablets: 10 mg, 25 mg

GUANETHIDINE
gwahn ETH i deen
TRADE NAME(S):
Ismelin
THERAPEUTIC CLASS:
Antihypertensive
GENERAL USES:
Hypertension
DOSAGE FORMS:
Tablets: 10 mg, 25 mg

GUANFACINE
GWAHN fa seen
TRADE NAME(S):
Intuniv, Tenex

THERAPEUTIC CLASS:
ADHD agent,
antihypertensive
GENERAL USES:
Hypertension, ADHD
DOSAGE FORMS:
Tablets: 1 mg, 2 mg;
Extended-release tablets:
1 mg, 2 mg, 3 mg, 4 mg

HALCINONIDE
hal SIN oh nide
TRADE NAME(S):
Halog, Halog-E
THERAPEUTIC CLASS:
Corticosteroid (topical)
GENERAL USES:
Various skin conditions
DOSAGE FORMS:
Ointment, Solution, and
Cream: 0.1%; Cream:
0.025%

HALOFANTRINE
ha loe FAN trin
TRADE NAME(S):
Halfan
THERAPEUTIC CLASS:
Antimalarial
GENERAL USES:
Malaria treatment
DOSAGE FORMS:
Tablets: 250 mg

HALOPERIDOL
ha loe PER i dole
TRADE NAME(S):
Haldol

THERAPEUTIC CLASS:
Antipsychotic
GENERAL USES:
Psychotic/behavioral
disorders, Tourette's
DOSAGE FORMS:
Tablets: 0.5 mg, 1 mg,
2 mg, 5 mg, 10 mg,
20 mg; Concentrated
solution: 2 mg/mL;
Injection: 5 mg, 50 mg,
100 mg, 250 mg, 500 mg

HALOPROGIN
ha loe PROE jin
TRADE NAME(S):
Halotex
THERAPEUTIC CLASS:
Antifungal (topical)
GENERAL USES:
Athlete's foot, jock itch,
ringworm, tinea versicolor
DOSAGE FORMS:
Cream and Solution: 1%

HEPARIN
HEP a rin
TRADE NAME(S):
Heparin
THERAPEUTIC CLASS:
Anticoagulant
GENERAL USES:
Prevention of blood clots
DOSAGE FORMS:
Various concentrations

HETASTARCH
HET a starch
TRADE NAME(S):
 Hespan
THERAPEUTIC CLASS:
 Plasma expander
GENERAL USES:
 Shock
DOSAGE FORMS:
 Injection: 30 g

HUMAN PAPILLOMAVIRUS (HPV) VACCINE
pap i LOE ma VYE rus vak SEEN
TRADE NAME(S):
 Gardasil, Cervarix
THERAPEUTIC CLASS:
 Vaccine
GENERAL USES:
 Prevention of HPV
DOSAGE FORMS:
 Injection: 0.5 mL (various HPV proteins)

HYALURONIDASE
hye al yoor ON i dase
TRADE NAME(S):
 Hydase, Amphadase
THERAPEUTIC CLASS:
 Enzyme
GENERAL USES:
 Increase absorption and dispersion of drugs

DOSAGE FORMS:
 Injection: 150 units, 300 units

HYALURONIDASE (OVINE)
hye al yoor ON i dase
TRADE NAME(S):
 Vitrase
THERAPEUTIC CLASS:
 Enzyme
GENERAL USES:
 Increase absorption of injected drugs
DOSAGE FORMS:
 Injection: 6200 units

HYDRALAZINE
hye DRAL a zeen
TRADE NAME(S):
 Apresoline
THERAPEUTIC CLASS:
 Antihypertensive
GENERAL USES:
 Hypertension
DOSAGE FORMS:
 Tablets: 10 mg, 25 mg, 50 mg, 100 mg; Injection: 20 mg

HYDRALAZINE/HCTZ
hye DRAL a zeen/hye droe klor oh THYE a zide
TRADE NAME(S):
 Apresazide
THERAPEUTIC CLASS:
 Antihypertensive/diuretic

GENERAL USES:
Hypertension

DOSAGE FORMS:
Tablets: 25 mg/25 mg,
50 mg/50 mg, 100 mg/
50 mg

HYDRALAZINE/
ISOSORBIDE DINITRATE
hye DRAL a zeen/eye soe
SOR bide dye NYE trate

TRADE NAME(S):
BiDil

THERAPEUTIC CLASS:
Antihypertensive/
antianginal

GENERAL USES:
Heart failure

DOSAGE FORMS:
Tablets: 37.5 mg/20 mg

HYDROCHLOROTHIAZIDE
hye droe klor oh THYE a zide

TRADE NAME(S):
Esidrix, HydroDIURIL,
Microzide, Oretic

THERAPEUTIC CLASS:
Diuretic

GENERAL USES:
CHF-related edema,
hypertension

DOSAGE FORMS:
Tablets: 25 mg, 50 mg,
100 mg; Capsules:
12.5 mg; Solution:
50 mg/5 mL

HYDROCODONE
HYE droe KOE done

TRADE NAME(S):
Zohydro ER

THERAPEUTIC CLASS:
Analgesic

GENERAL USES:
Pain

DOSAGE FORMS:
Extended-release
capsules: 10 mg, 15 mg,
20 mg, 30 mg, 40 mg,
50 mg

HYDROCODONE/
ACETAMINOPHEN
hye droe KOE done/a seet a
MIN oh fen

TRADE NAME(S):
Anexsia, Hycet, Lorcet,
Lortab, Vicodin, Xodol,
Zamicet, Zolvit

THERAPEUTIC CLASS:
Analgesic

GENERAL USES:
Pain

DOSAGE FORMS:
Tablets: 5 mg/325 mg, 7.5
mg/325 mg, 10 mg/325
mg; Solution (per 15 mL):
7.5 mg/325 mg, 10 mg/
325 mg, 10 mg/300 mg

HYDROCODONE/
CHLORPHENIRAMINE
HYE droe KOE done/klor fen
IR a meen

Trade Name(s):
Tussionex, Vituz

Therapeutic Class:
Analgesic/Antihistamine

General Uses:
Cough and cold

Dosage Forms:
Extended-release suspension: 10 mg/8 mg per 5 mL; Solution: 5 mg/4 mg per 5 mL

HYDROCODONE/ IBUPROFEN
HYE droe KOE done/eye byoo PROE fen

Trade Name(s):
Ibudone, Reprexain, Vicoprofen

Therapeutic Class:
Analgesic

General Uses:
Pain

Dosage Forms:
Tablets: 2.5 mg/200 mg, 5 mg/200 mg, 7.5 mg/ 200 mg, 10 mg/200 mg

HYDROCORTISONE (ORAL)
hye droe KOR ti sone

Trade Name(s):
Cortef

Therapeutic Class:
Glucocorticoid

General Uses:
Endocrine, skin, blood disorders

Dosage Forms:
Tablets: 5 mg, 10 mg, 20 mg

HYDROCORTISONE (TOPICAL)
hye droe KOR ti sone

Trade Name(s):
Hycort, Cort-Dome, Dermacort, many others

Therapeutic Class:
Corticosteroid (topical)

General Uses:
Various skin conditions

Dosage Forms:
Ointment, Lotion, and Cream: 0.5%, 1%, 2.5%; Lotion: 2%; Gel, Solution, and Spray: 1%

HYDROCORTISONE ACETATE
hye droe KOR ti sone

Trade Name(s):
Hydrocortone Acetate

Therapeutic Class:
Glucocorticoid

General Uses:
Endocrine, skin, blood disorders

Dosage Forms:
Injection: 125 mg, 250 mg, 500 mg

**HYDROCORTISONE
SODIUM SUCCINATE**
hye droe KOR ti sone
TRADE NAME(S):
Solu-Cortef, A-Hydrocort
THERAPEUTIC CLASS:
Glucocorticoid
GENERAL USES:
Endocrine, skin, blood
disorders
DOSAGE FORMS:
Injection: 100 mg,
250 mg, 500 mg,
1000 mg

HYDROMORPHONE
HYE droe MOR fone
TRADE NAME(S):
Dilaudid, Dilaudid-HP,
Exalgo
THERAPEUTIC CLASS:
Analgesic (narcotic)
GENERAL USES:
Pain
DOSAGE FORMS:
Injection: 10 mg, 50 mg,
250 mg, 500 mg;
Solution: 5 mg/5 mL;
Tablets: 2 mg, 4 mg,
8 mg; Extended-release
tablets: 8 mg, 12 mg, 16
mg, 32 mg

**HYDROXY-
AMPHETAMINE**
HYE droks ee am FET a
meen

TRADE NAME(S):
Paredrine
THERAPEUTIC CLASS:
Ocular agent
GENERAL USES:
Pupil dilation
DOSAGE FORMS:
Ophthalmic solution: 1%

**HYDROXY-
CHLOROQUINE**
hye droks ee KLOR oh kwin
TRADE NAME(S):
Plaquenil
THERAPEUTIC CLASS:
Antirheumatic agent
GENERAL USES:
Rheumatoid arthritis,
systemic lupus
erythematosus
DOSAGE FORMS:
Tablets: 200 mg

**HYDROXYPRO-
GESTERONE CAPROATE**
hye DROKS ee proe JES ter
one KAP roe ate
TRADE NAME(S):
Makena
THERAPEUTIC CLASS:
Progestin
GENERAL USES:
Reduce risk of preterm
birth
DOSAGE FORMS:
Injection: 1250 mg

HYDROXYZINE
hye DROKS i zeen
TRADE NAME(S):
Atarax, Vistaril
THERAPEUTIC CLASS:
Antihistamine
GENERAL USES:
Itching, sedation
DOSAGE FORMS:
Tablets: 10 mg, 25 mg,
50 mg, 100 mg; Capsules:
25 mg, 50 mg, 100 mg;
Syrup: 10 mg/5 mL;
Suspension: 25 mg/5 mL;
Injection: 25 mg, 50 mg

IBANDRONATE
eye BAN droh nate
TRADE NAME(S):
Boniva
THERAPEUTIC CLASS:
Bisphosphonate
GENERAL USES:
Postmenopausal
osteoporosis
DOSAGE FORMS:
Injection: 3 mg;
Tablets: 2.5 mg,
150 mg

IBRITUMOMAB
ib ri TYOO mo mab
TRADE NAME(S):
Zevalin
THERAPEUTIC CLASS:
Monoclonal antibody
GENERAL USES:
Non-Hodgkin's lymphoma

DOSAGE FORMS:
Injection: 3.2 mg

IBRUTINIB
eye BROO ti nib
TRADE NAME(S):
Imbruvica
THERAPEUTIC CLASS:
Antineoplastic
GENERAL USES:
Mantle cell lymphoma,
CLL
DOSAGE FORMS:
Capsules: 140 mg

IBUPROFEN
EYE byoo PROE fen
TRADE NAME(S):
Caldolor, Motrin, Advil,
Nuprin, many others
THERAPEUTIC CLASS:
Analgesic, antipyretic,
anti-inflammatory
GENERAL USES:
Pain, fever, arthritis
DOSAGE FORMS:
Tablets: 100 mg, 200 mg,
300 mg, 400 mg, 600 mg,
800 mg; Chewable
tablets: 50 mg, 100 mg;
Capsules: 200 mg; Liquid
or Suspension: 100 mg/
5 mL; Suspension:
100 mg/2.5 mL; Drops:
40 mg/mL; Injection:
400 mg, 800 mg

ICATIBANT ACETATE
eye KAT i bant AS e tate
TRADE NAME(S):
Firazyr
THERAPEUTIC CLASS:
Hematological agent
GENERAL USES:
Hereditary angioedema
DOSAGE FORMS:
Injection: 30 mg

ICOSAPENT ETHYL
eye KOE sa pent ETH il
TRADE NAME(S):
Vascepa
THERAPEUTIC CLASS:
Fish oil
GENERAL USES:
Hypertriglyceridemia
DOSAGE FORMS:
Capsules: 1 g

IDELALISIB
eye del a LIS ib
TRADE NAME(S):
Zydelig
THERAPEUTIC CLASS:
Antineoplastic
GENERAL USES:
CLL, various lymphomas
DOSAGE FORMS:
Tablets: 100 mg, 150 mg

IDOXURIDINE
eye doks YOOR i deen
TRADE NAME(S):
Herplex

THERAPEUTIC CLASS:
Ocular agent (antiviral)
GENERAL USES:
Ocular herpes
infections
DOSAGE FORMS:
Ophthalmic solution: 0.1%

IDURSULFASE
eye dur SUL fase
TRADE NAME(S):
Elaprase
THERAPEUTIC CLASS:
Enzyme
GENERAL USES:
Hunter syndrome
DOSAGE FORMS:
Injection: 5 mL

ILOPERIDONE
EYE loe PER i done
TRADE NAME(S):
Fanapt
THERAPEUTIC CLASS:
Antipsychotic
GENERAL USES:
Schizophrenia
DOSAGE FORMS:
Tablets: 1 mg, 2 mg,
4 mg, 6 mg, 8 mg, 10 mg,
12 mg

ILOPROST
EYE loe prost
TRADE NAME(S):
Ventavis
THERAPEUTIC CLASS:
Antihypertensive

GENERAL USES:
Pulmonary hypertension
DOSAGE FORMS:
Inhalation: 10 mcg,
20 mcg

IMATINIB
eye MAT eh nib
TRADE NAME(S):
Gleevec
THERAPEUTIC CLASS:
Antineoplastic
GENERAL USES:
CLL, GI stromal tumors,
ALL
DOSAGE FORMS:
Capsules: 100 mg

IMIPENEM/CILASTATIN
i mi PEN em/sye la STAT in
TRADE NAME(S):
Primaxin
THERAPEUTIC CLASS:
Anti-infective
GENERAL USES:
Bacterial infections
DOSAGE FORMS:
Injection: 250 mg/250 mg
500 mg/500 mg,
750 mg/750 mg

IMIPRAMINE HCL
im IP ra meen
TRADE NAME(S):
Tofranil
THERAPEUTIC CLASS:
Antidepressant

GENERAL USES:
Depression,
childhood
bedwetting
DOSAGE FORMS:
Tablets: 10 mg, 25 mg,
50 mg

IMIPRAMINE PAMOATE
im IP ra meen
TRADE NAME(S):
Tofranil-PM
THERAPEUTIC CLASS:
Antidepressant
GENERAL USES:
Depression
DOSAGE FORMS:
Capsules: 75 mg, 100 mg,
125 mg, 150 mg

IMIQUIMOD
i mi KWI mod
TRADE NAME(S):
Aldara, Zyclara
THERAPEUTIC CLASS:
Immunomodulator
(topical)
GENERAL USES:
Actinic keratosis, genital
and anal warts, basal cell
carcinoma
DOSAGE FORMS:
Cream: 3.75%, 5%

INCOBOTULINUM-
TOXINA
INK oh BOT yoo li num TOKS
in AY

TRADE NAME(S):
Xeomin

THERAPEUTIC CLASS:
Toxoid

GENERAL USES:
Cervical dystonia, eyelid tics

DOSAGE FORMS:
Injection: 50 units, 100 units

INDACATEROL MALEATE
IN da KAT er ol MAL ee ate

TRADE NAME(S):
Arcapta Neohaler

THERAPEUTIC CLASS:
Bronchodilator

GENERAL USES:
COPD

DOSAGE FORMS:
Inhalation powder (capsules): 75 mcg

INDAPAMIDE
in DAP a mide

TRADE NAME(S):
Lozol

THERAPEUTIC CLASS:
Diuretic

GENERAL USES:
CHF, hypertension

DOSAGE FORMS:
Tablets: 1.25 mg, 2.5 mg

INDINAVIR
in DIN a veer

TRADE NAME(S):
Crixivan

THERAPEUTIC CLASS:
Antiviral

GENERAL USES:
HIV infection

DOSAGE FORMS:
Capsules: 100 mg, 200 mg, 333 mg, 400 mg

INDOMETHACIN
in doe METH a sin

TRADE NAME(S):
Indocin, Indocin ER, Indocin SR, Tivorbex

THERAPEUTIC CLASS:
Anti-inflammatory/ analgesic

GENERAL USES:
Various arthritis conditions, pain

DOSAGE FORMS:
Capsules: 20 mg, 25 mg, 40 mg, 50 mg; Sustained-release capsules: 75 mg; Suspension: 25 mg/5 mL

INFLIXIMAB
in FLIKS i mab

TRADE NAME(S):
Remicade

THERAPEUTIC CLASS:
Monoclonal antibody

GENERAL USES:
Crohn's disease, various arthritis syndromes, ulcerative colitis, psoriasis, psoriatic arthritis

DOSAGE FORMS:
Injection: 100 mg

INFLUENZA VIRUS VACCINE
in floo EN za VYE rus vak SEEN
TRADE NAME(S):
Flublok, Flucelvax
THERAPEUTIC CLASS:
Vaccine
GENERAL USES:
Prevent infection with influenza virus
DOSAGE FORMS:
Injection: 0.5 mL

INFLUENZA VIRUS VACCINE, LIVE (INTRANASAL)
in floo EN za VYE rus vak SEEN
TRADE NAME(S):
FluMist
THERAPEUTIC CLASS:
Vaccine
GENERAL USES:
Prevention of influenza
DOSAGE FORMS:
Nasal spray: 0.5 mL

INGENOL MEBUTATE
IN je nol MEB yoo tate
TRADE NAME(S):
Picato
THERAPEUTIC CLASS:
Dermatologic agent
GENERAL USES:
Actinic keratosis
DOSAGE FORMS:
Gel: 0.015%, 0.05%

INSULIN, ASPART
IN su lin AS part
TRADE NAME(S):
NovoLog
THERAPEUTIC CLASS:
Antidiabetic
GENERAL USES:
Diabetes
DOSAGE FORMS:
Injection: 100 units/mL

INSULIN, DETEMIR
IN su lin DE te meer
TRADE NAME(S):
Levemir
THERAPEUTIC CLASS:
Antidiabetic
GENERAL USES:
Diabetes
DOSAGE FORMS:
Injection: 100 units/mL

INSULIN, GLARGINE
IN su lin GLAR jeen
TRADE NAME(S):
Lantus
THERAPEUTIC CLASS:
Antidiabetic
GENERAL USES:
Diabetes
DOSAGE FORMS:
Injection: 100 units/mL

INSULIN, GLULISINE
IN su lin gloo LIS een
TRADE NAME(S):
Apidra
THERAPEUTIC CLASS:
Antidiabetic
GENERAL USES:
Diabetes
DOSAGE FORMS:
Injection: 100 units/mL

INSULIN, HUMAN (rDNA)
IN su lin
TRADE NAME(S):
Afrezza
THERAPEUTIC CLASS:
Antidiabetic
GENERAL USES:
Diabetes
DOSAGE FORMS:
Oral inhalation:
4 units, 8 units

INSULIN, ISOPHANE SUSPENSION
IN su lin EYE soe fane
TRADE NAME(S):
Novolin N, Humulin N
THERAPEUTIC CLASS:
Antidiabetic
GENERAL USES:
Diabetes
DOSAGE FORMS:
Injection: 100 units/mL

INSULIN, ISOPHANE SUSPENSION AND INSULIN REGULAR
IN su lin
TRADE NAME(S):
Humulin 50/50, Novolin 70/30, Humulin 70/30
THERAPEUTIC CLASS:
Antidiabetic
GENERAL USES:
Diabetes
DOSAGE FORMS:
Injection: 100 units/mL

INSULIN, LISPRO
IN su lin LYE sproe
TRADE NAME(S):
Humalog
THERAPEUTIC CLASS:
Antidiabetic
GENERAL USES:
Diabetes
DOSAGE FORMS:
Injection: 100 units/mL

INSULIN, LISPRO PROTAMINE SUSPENSION AND INSULIN LISPRO
IN su lin
TRADE NAME(S):
Humalog 75/25
THERAPEUTIC CLASS:
Antidiabetic
GENERAL USES:
Diabetes
DOSAGE FORMS:
Injection: 100 units/mL

INSULIN, REGULAR
IN su lin
TRADE NAME(S):
Novolin R, Humulin R
THERAPEUTIC CLASS:
Antidiabetic
GENERAL USES:
Diabetes
DOSAGE FORMS:
Injection: 100 units/mL

INSULIN, ZINC SUSPENSION
IN su lin
TRADE NAME(S):
Humulin L
THERAPEUTIC CLASS:
Antidiabetic
GENERAL USES:
Diabetes
DOSAGE FORMS:
Injection: 100 units/mL

INSULIN, ZINC SUSPENSION, EXTENDED
IN su lin
TRADE NAME(S):
Humulin U
THERAPEUTIC CLASS:
Antidiabetic
GENERAL USES:
Diabetes
DOSAGE FORMS:
Injection: 100 units/mL

INTERFERON ALFA-2a
in ter FEER on
TRADE NAME(S):
Roferon-A
THERAPEUTIC CLASS:
Immune modulator
GENERAL USES:
Leukemia, AIDS sarcoma
DOSAGE FORMS:
Injection: 3 million international units (IU), 6 million IU, 9 million IU, 18 million IU, 36 million IU

INTERFERON ALFA-2b
in ter FEER on
TRADE NAME(S):
Intron-A
THERAPEUTIC CLASS:
Immune modulator
GENERAL USES:
Leukemia, AIDS sarcoma, hepatitis B, C (chronic)
DOSAGE FORMS:
Injection: 3 million international units (IU), 5 million IU, 10 million IU, 18 million IU, 25 million IU, 50 million IU

INTERFERON BETA-1a
in ter FEER on
TRADE NAME(S):
Avonex, Rebif
THERAPEUTIC CLASS:
Immune modulator
GENERAL USES:
Multiple sclerosis

DOSAGE FORMS:
  Injection: 6.6 million international units (33 mcg)

INTERFERON BETA-1b
in ter FEER on
TRADE NAME(S):
  Betaseron, Extavia
THERAPEUTIC CLASS:
  Immune modulator
GENERAL USES:
  Multiple sclerosis
DOSAGE FORMS:
  Injection: 0.3 mg

IOBENGUANE SULFATE I 123
eye oh BEN gwane
TRADE NAME(S):
  AdreView
THERAPEUTIC CLASS:
  Radiopaque agent
GENERAL USES:
  Diagnosis of pheochromocytoma and other cancers
DOSAGE FORMS:
  Injection: 10 mCi/5 mL

IODOQUINOL
eye oh doe KWIN ole
TRADE NAME(S):
  Yodoxin
THERAPEUTIC CLASS:
  Antituberculosis agent
GENERAL USES:
  Tuberculosis

DOSAGE FORMS:
  Tablets: 210 mg, 650 mg; Powder: 25 g

IOFLUPANE I 123
EYE oh FLOO pane
TRADE NAME(S):
  DaTscan
THERAPEUTIC CLASS:
  Radiopaque agent
GENERAL USES:
  Brain imaging
DOSAGE FORMS:
  Injection: 185 MBq (5 mCi)

IPILIMUMAB
IP i LIM yoo mab
TRADE NAME(S):
  Yervoy
THERAPEUTIC CLASS:
  Antineoplastic
GENERAL USES:
  Metastatic melanoma
DOSAGE FORMS:
  Injection: 50 mg, 200 mg

IPRATROPIUM
i pra TROE pee um
TRADE NAME(S):
  Atrovent
THERAPEUTIC CLASS:
  Bronchodilator
GENERAL USES:
  Bronchospasm, asthma
DOSAGE FORMS:
  Inhalation solution: 0.02%; Inhaler: 18 mcg/

inhalation; Nasal spray:
0.03%, 0.06%

IPRATROPIUM/ ALBUTEROL
i pra TROE pee um/al BYOO ter ole

TRADE NAME(S):
Combivent, Combivent Respimat

THERAPEUTIC CLASS:
Bronchodilator

GENERAL USES:
Bronchospasm

DOSAGE FORMS:
Inhaler: 18 mcg/103 mcg/ inhalation, 20 mg/ 100 mcg/inhalation

IRBESARTAN
ir be SAR tan

TRADE NAME(S):
Avapro

THERAPEUTIC CLASS:
Antihypertensive

GENERAL USES:
Hypertension, diabetic nephropathy

DOSAGE FORMS:
Tablets: 75 mg, 150 mg, 300 mg

IRBESARTAN/HCTZ
ir be SAR tan/hye droe klor oh THYE a zide

TRADE NAME(S):
Avalide

THERAPEUTIC CLASS:
Antihypertensive/ diuretic

GENERAL USES:
Hypertension

DOSAGE FORMS:
Tablets: 150 mg/12.5 mg, 300 mg/12.5 mg

ISOCARBOXAZID
eye so kar BOKS a zid

TRADE NAME(S):
Marplan

THERAPEUTIC CLASS:
Antidepressant

GENERAL USES:
Depression

DOSAGE FORMS:
Tablets: 10 mg

ISOETHARINE
eye soe ETH a reen

TRADE NAME(S):
Bronkosol

THERAPEUTIC CLASS:
Bronchodilator

GENERAL USES:
Bronchospasm, asthma

DOSAGE FORMS:
Inhalation solution: 1%

ISONIAZID
eye soe NYE a zid

TRADE NAME(S):
Laniazid, Nydrazid

THERAPEUTIC CLASS:
Antituberculosis agent

GENERAL USES:
Tuberculosis

DOSAGE FORMS:
Tablets: 50 mg, 100 mg,
300 mg; Syrup: 50 mg/
5 mL; Injection: 1 g

ISOPROTERENOL
eye soe proe TER e nole

TRADE NAME(S):
Medihaler-Iso

THERAPEUTIC CLASS:
Bronchodilator

GENERAL USES:
Bronchospasm,
asthma

DOSAGE FORMS:
Inhaler: 80 mcg/inhalation

ISOSORBIDE DINITRATE
eye soe SOR bide dye NYE
trate

TRADE NAME(S):
Isordil, Sorbitrate

THERAPEUTIC CLASS:
Antianginal

GENERAL USES:
Angina

DOSAGE FORMS:
Tablets: 5 mg, 10 mg,
20 mg, 30 mg, 40 mg;
Sustained-release tablets
and capsules: 40 mg;
Sublingual tablets:
2.5 mg, 5 mg, 10 mg;
Chewable tablets: 5 mg,
10 mg

ISOSORBIDE MONONITRATE
eye soe SOR bide mon oh
NYE trate

TRADE NAME(S):
Ismo, Monoket,
Imdur

THERAPEUTIC CLASS:
Antianginal

GENERAL USES:
Angina

DOSAGE FORMS:
Tablets: 10 mg, 20 mg;
Extended-release tablets:
30 mg, 60 mg, 120 mg

ISOTRETINOIN
eye soe TRET i noyn

TRADE NAME(S):
Absorica, Accutane

THERAPEUTIC CLASS:
Retinoid

GENERAL USES:
Severe cystic acne

DOSAGE FORMS:
Capsules: 10 mg, 20 mg,
30 mg, 40 mg

ISRADIPINE
iz RA di peen

TRADE NAME(S):
DynaCirc CR,
DynaCirc

THERAPEUTIC CLASS:
Antihypertensive

GENERAL USES:
Hypertension

DOSAGE FORMS:
Capsules: 2.5 mg, 5 mg;
Controlled-release tablets:
5 mg, 10 mg

ITRACONAZOLE
i tra KOE na zole
TRADE NAME(S):
Sporanox
THERAPEUTIC CLASS:
Antifungal
GENERAL USES:
Fungal infections
DOSAGE FORMS:
Capsules: 100 mg;
Solution: 10 mg/mL;
Injection: 10 mg

IVACAFTOR
EYE va KAF tor
TRADE NAME(S):
Kalydeco
THERAPEUTIC CLASS:
Cystic fibrosis agent
GENERAL USES:
Cystic fibrosis
DOSAGE FORMS:
Tablets: 150 mg

IVERMECTIN (ORAL)
EYE ver MEK tin
TRADE NAME(S):
Stromectol
THERAPEUTIC CLASS:
Anthelmintic
GENERAL USES:
GI parasite infections

DOSAGE FORMS:
Tablets: 3 mg

IVERMECTIN (TOPICAL)
EYE ver MEK tin
TRADE NAME(S):
Sklice
THERAPEUTIC CLASS:
Pediculicide
GENERAL USES:
Head lice
DOSAGE FORMS:
Lotion: 0.5%

IXABEPILONE
iks ab EP i lone
TRADE NAME(S):
Ixempra
THERAPEUTIC CLASS:
Antineoplastic
GENERAL USES:
Breast cancer
DOSAGE FORMS:
Injection: 15 mg,
45 mg

KANAMYCIN
kan a MYE sin
TRADE NAME(S):
Kantrex
THERAPEUTIC CLASS:
Anti-infective
GENERAL USES:
Bacterial infections
DOSAGE FORMS:
Injection: 150 mg, 1 g,
2 g, 3 g

KETOCONAZOLE
kee toe KOE na zole
TRADE NAME(S):
Nizoral, Xolegel
THERAPEUTIC CLASS:
Antifungal (oral and topical)
GENERAL USES:
Fungal infections
DOSAGE FORMS:
Tablets: 200 mg; Shampoo, Gel, and Cream: 2%

KETOPROFEN
kee toe PROE fen
TRADE NAME(S):
Orudis KT, Actron, Orudis, Oruvail
THERAPEUTIC CLASS:
Anti-inflammatory/analgesic
GENERAL USES:
Osteoarthritis, rheumatoid arthritis, pain
DOSAGE FORMS:
Capsules: 12.5 mg, 25 mg, 50 mg, 75 mg; Extended-release capsules: 100 mg, 150 mg, 200 mg

KETOROLAC
kee toe ROLE ak
TRADE NAME(S):
Toradol
THERAPEUTIC CLASS:
Anti-inflammatory/analgesic
GENERAL USES:
Severe acute pain (short-term therapy)
DOSAGE FORMS:
Tablets: 10 mg; Injection: 15 mg, 30 mg, 60 mg

KETOROLAC (OCULAR)
kee toe ROLE ak
TRADE NAME(S):
Acular, Acuvail
THERAPEUTIC CLASS:
Ocular agent
GENERAL USES:
Allergic conjunctivitis, post-op pain
DOSAGE FORMS:
Ophthalmic solution: 0.45%, 0.5%

KETOROLAC TROMETHAMINE (NASAL)
kee toe ROLE ak
TRADE NAME(S):
Sprix
THERAPEUTIC CLASS:
Nasal agent
GENERAL USES:
Pain
DOSAGE FORMS:
Nasal spray: 15.75 mg/spray

KETOROLAC/ PHENYLEPHRINE
kee toe ROLE ak/fen ill EFF rin

TRADE NAME(S):
Omidria

THERAPEUTIC CLASS:
Anti-inflammatory/ sympathomimetic

GENERAL USES:
Eye surgery, pain

DOSAGE FORMS:
Solution: 1%/0.3%

KETOTIFEN
kee toe TYE fen

TRADE NAME(S):
Zaditor

THERAPEUTIC CLASS:
Ocular agent

GENERAL USES:
Allergic conjunctivitis

DOSAGE FORMS:
Ophthalmic solution: 0.025%

LABETALOL
la BET a lole

TRADE NAME(S):
Normodyne, Trandate

THERAPEUTIC CLASS:
Antihypertensive

GENERAL USES:
Hypertension

DOSAGE FORMS:
Tablets: 100 mg, 200 mg, 300 mg

LACOSAMIDE
la KOE sa mide

TRADE NAME(S):
Vimpat

THERAPEUTIC CLASS:
Anticonvulsant

GENERAL USES:
Seizures

DOSAGE FORMS:
Oral solution: 10 mg/mL; Injection: 200 mg/20 mL; Tablets: 50 mg, 100 mg, 150 mg, 200 mg

LAMIVUDINE (3TC)
la MI vyoo deen

TRADE NAME(S):
Epivir, Epivir-HBV

THERAPEUTIC CLASS:
Antiviral

GENERAL USES:
HIV infection

DOSAGE FORMS:
Tablets: 100 mg, 150 mg; Solution: 5 mg/mL, 10 mg/mL

LAMIVUDINE/ NEVIRAPINE/ ZIDOVUDINE
la MI vyoo deen/ne VYE ra peen/zye DOE vyoo deen

TRADE NAME(S):
Lamivudine/Nevirapine/ Zidovudine

THERAPEUTIC CLASS:
Antiviral

GENERAL USES:
  HIV infection
DOSAGE FORMS:
  Tablets (for oral
  suspension): 30 mg/
  50 mg/60 mg

LAMIVUDINE/
ZIDOVUDINE
la MI vyoo deen/zye DOE
vyoo deen
TRADE NAME(S):
  Combivir
THERAPEUTIC CLASS:
  Antiviral
GENERAL USES:
  HIV infection
DOSAGE FORMS:
  Tablets: 150 mg/300 mg

LAMOTRIGINE
la MOE tri jeen
TRADE NAME(S):
  Lamictal, Lamictal ODT,
  Lamictal XR
THERAPEUTIC CLASS:
  Anticonvulsant
GENERAL USES:
  Seizures, bipolar disorder
DOSAGE FORMS:
  Extended-release tablets
  and Tablets: 25 mg,
  100 mg, 150 mg, 200 mg;
  Chewable tablets: 5 mg,
  25 mg; Orally
  disintegrating tablets:
  25 mg, 50 mg, 100 mg,
  200 mg

LANREOTIDE
lan REE oh tide
TRADE NAME(S):
  Somatuline Depot
THERAPEUTIC CLASS:
  Hormone
GENERAL USES:
  Acromegaly
DOSAGE FORMS:
  Injection: 60 mg, 90 mg,
  120 mg

LANSOPRAZOLE
lan SOE pra zole
TRADE NAME(S):
  Prevacid, Prevacid 24-
  Hour
THERAPEUTIC CLASS:
  Gastric acid secretion
  inhibitor
GENERAL USES:
  Duodenal ulcer,
  GERD
DOSAGE FORMS:
  Delayed-release capsules
  and suspension: 15 mg,
  30 mg

LANSOPRAZOLE/
NAPROXEN
lan SOE pra zole/na PROKS
en
TRADE NAME(S):
  Prevacid/NapraPAC
THERAPEUTIC CLASS:
  Gastric acid secretion
  inhibitor/NSAID

GENERAL USES:
Arthritis in patients at risk
for gastric ulcers

DOSAGE FORMS:
Tablets: 15 mg/375 mg,
15 mg/500 mg

LANTHANUM CARBONATE
LAN tha num

TRADE NAME(S):
Fosrenol

THERAPEUTIC CLASS:
Phosphate binder

GENERAL USES:
End-stage renal disease

DOSAGE FORMS:
Tablets: 500 mg, 750 mg,
1000 mg; Oral powder:
750 mg, 1000 mg

LAPATINIB
la PA ti nib

TRADE NAME(S):
Tykerb

THERAPEUTIC CLASS:
Antineoplastic

GENERAL USES:
Breast cancer

DOSAGE FORMS:
Tablets: 250 mg

LARONIDASE
lair OH ni days

TRADE NAME(S):
Aldurazyme

THERAPEUTIC CLASS:
Enzyme

GENERAL USES:
Mucopolysaccharidosis I

DOSAGE FORMS:
Injection: 2.9 mg

LATANOPROST
la TA noe prost

TRADE NAME(S):
Xalatan

THERAPEUTIC CLASS:
Ocular agent

GENERAL USES:
Glaucoma/ocular
hypertension

DOSAGE FORMS:
Ophthalmic solution:
0.005%

LEDIPASVIR/ SOFOSBUVIR
le DIP as veer/soe FOS
byoo veer

TRADE NAME(S):
Harvoni

THERAPEUTIC CLASS:
Antiviral

GENERAL CLASS:
Hepatitis C virus

DOSAGE FORMS:
Tablets: 90 mg/400 mg

LEFLUNOMIDE
le FLOO noh mide

TRADE NAME(S):
Arava

THERAPEUTIC CLASS:
Antirheumatic

GENERAL USES:
Rheumatoid arthritis
DOSAGE FORMS:
Tablets: 10 mg, 20 mg, 100 mg

LENALIDOMIDE
le na LID oh mide
TRADE NAME(S):
Revlimid
THERAPEUTIC CLASS:
Immunologic agent
GENERAL USES:
Myelodysplastic syndrome, lymphoma
DOSAGE FORMS:
Capsules: 5 mg, 10 mg

LEPIRUDIN
le PEER u din
TRADE NAME(S):
Refludan
THERAPEUTIC CLASS:
Anticoagulant
GENERAL USES:
Heparin-induced thrombocytopenia
DOSAGE FORMS:
Injection: 50 mg

LETROZOLE
LET roe zole
TRADE NAME(S):
Femara
THERAPEUTIC CLASS:
Antineoplastic
GENERAL USES:
Breast cancer

DOSAGE FORMS:
Tablets: 2.5 mg

LEUPROLIDE ACETATE/ NORETHINDRONE ACETATE
loo PRO lide/nor eth IN drone
TRADE NAME(S):
Lupaneta Pack
THERAPEUTIC CLASS:
Endometrial hyperplasia agent
GENERAL USES:
Endometriosis
DOSAGE FORMS:
Leuprolide acetate depot suspension: 3.75 mg/ norethindrone acetate tablets: 5 mg

LEVALBUTEROL
lev al BYOO ter ol
TRADE NAME(S):
Xopenox, Xopenox HFA
THERAPEUTIC CLASS:
Bronchodilator
GENERAL USES:
Bronchospasm
DOSAGE FORMS:
Solution for inhalation: 0.31 mg/3 mL, 0.63 mg/ 3 mL, 1.25 mg/3 mL; Oral aerosol: 45 mcg/ actuation; Concentrate: 1.25 mg/0.5 mL

LEVETIRACETAM

lee ve tye RA se tam

TRADE NAME(S):
Keppra, Keppra IV, Keppra XR

THERAPEUTIC CLASS:
Anticonvulsant

GENERAL USES:
Partial seizures

DOSAGE FORMS:
Extended-release tablets: 500 mg, 750 mg; Tablets: 250 mg, 500 mg, 750 mg, 1000 mg; Oral solution: 100 mg/mL; Injection: 500 mg

LEVOBETAXOLOL

lee voe be TAKS oh lol

TRADE NAME(S):
Betaxon

THERAPEUTIC CLASS:
Ocular agent

GENERAL USES:
Open-angle glaucoma, ocular hypertension

DOSAGE FORMS:
Ophthalmic suspension: 0.5%

LEVOBUNOLOL

lee voe BYOO noe lole

TRADE NAME(S):
AKBeta, Betagan

THERAPEUTIC CLASS:
Ocular agent

GENERAL USES:
Glaucoma/ocular hypertension

DOSAGE FORMS:
Ophthalmic solution: 0.25%, 0.5%

LEVOCABASTINE

LEE voe kab as teen

TRADE NAME(S):
Livostin

THERAPEUTIC CLASS:
Ocular agent

GENERAL USES:
Allergic conjunctivitis

DOSAGE FORMS:
Ophthalmic suspension: 0.05%

LEVOCETIRIZINE

lee voe se TIR i zeen

TRADE NAME(S):
Xyzal

THERAPEUTIC CLASS:
Antihistamine

GENERAL USES:
Chronic hives, allergies

DOSAGE FORMS:
Tablets: 5 mg; Oral solution: 0.5 mg/mL

LEVODOPA/ CARBIDOPA

lee voe DOE pa/kar bi DOE pa

TRADE NAME(S):
Sinemet, Sinemet CR,

Parcopa
THERAPEUTIC CLASS:
Antiparkinson agent
GENERAL USES:
Parkinson's disease
DOSAGE FORMS:
Tablets: 100 mg/10 mg,
100 mg/25 mg, 250 mg/
25 mg; Sustained-release
tablets: 100 mg/
25 mg, 200 mg/
50 mg

LEVOFLOXACIN
lee voe FLOKS a sin
TRADE NAME(S):
Levaquin
THERAPEUTIC CLASS:
Anti-infective
GENERAL USES:
Bacterial infections
DOSAGE FORMS:
Tablets: 250 mg, 500 mg;
Injection: 250 mg,
500 mg, 750 mg; Oral
solution: 25 mg/mL

LEVOLEUCOVORIN
lee voe LOO koe VOE rin
TRADE NAME(S):
Fusilev
THERAPEUTIC CLASS:
Folate analog
GENERAL USES:
Methotrexate toxicity
DOSAGE FORMS:
Injection: 50 mg

LEVOMILNACIPRAN
LEE voe mil NA si pran
TRADE NAME(S):
Fetzima
THERAPEUTIC CLASS:
Antidepressant
GENERAL USES:
Depression
DOSAGE FORMS:
Extended-release
capsules: 20 mg, 40 mg,
80 mg, 120 mg

LEVONORGESTREL
LEE voe nor jes trel
TRADE NAME(S):
Plan B, Skyla, Mirena
THERAPEUTIC CLASS:
Contraceptive
(emergency)
GENERAL USES:
Emergency contraception,
contraception
DOSAGE FORMS:
Intrauterine device: 13.5 mg,
52 mg; Tablets: 0.75 mg;

LEVOTHYROXINE
lee voe thye ROKS een
TRADE NAME(S):
Synthroid, Levothroid,
Levo-T, Levoxyl
THERAPEUTIC CLASS:
Hormone (thyroid)
GENERAL USES:
Hypothyroidism
DOSAGE FORMS:
Tablets: 25 mcg, 50 mcg,

75 mcg, 88 mcg,
100 mcg, 112 mcg,
125 mcg, 137 mcg,
150 mcg, 175 mcg,
200 mcg, 300 mcg;
Injection: 200 mcg,
500 mcg

L-GLUTAMINE
L GLOO ta meen
TRADE NAME(S):
NutreStore
THERAPEUTIC CLASS:
Amino acid
GENERAL USES:
Short bowel syndrome
DOSAGE FORMS:
Powder packet for oral
solution: 5 g

LIDOCAINE
LYE doe kane
TRADE NAME(S):
Xylocaine
THERAPEUTIC CLASS:
Antiarrhythmic
GENERAL USES:
Arrhythmias
DOSAGE FORMS:
Injection: 50 mg, 200 mg,
300 mg, 400 mg, 500 mg,
1 g, 2 g, 4 g

LIDOCAINE
LYE doe kane
TRADE NAME(S):
Zingo

THERAPEUTIC CLASS:
Anesthetic, local
GENERAL USES:
Venipuncture pain
DOSAGE FORMS:
Injection: 0.5 mg

LIDOCAINE
(TRANSDERMAL)
LYE doe kane
TRADE NAME(S):
Lidoderm
THERAPEUTIC CLASS:
Anesthetic, local
GENERAL USES:
Postherpetic neuralgia
DOSAGE FORMS:
Cream: 7%/7%;
Patch: 5%

LIDOCAINE/
TETRACAINE
LYE doe kane/TET
ra kane
TRADE NAME(S):
Synera, Pliaglis
THERAPEUTIC CLASS:
Anesthetic
GENERAL USES:
Topical anesthesia
DOSAGE FORMS:
Patch: 70 mg/70 mg;
Cream: 7%/7%

LINACLOTIDE
LIN a CLO tide
TRADE NAME(S):
Linzess

THERAPEUTIC CLASS:
GI agent
GENERAL USES:
Irritable bowel
(constipation), chronic
constipation
DOSAGE FORMS:
Capsules: 145 mcg,
290 mcg

LINAGLIPTIN
LIN a GLIP tin
TRADE NAME(S):
Tradjenta
THERAPEUTIC CLASS:
Antidiabetic
GENERAL USES:
Diabetes (type 2)
DOSAGE FORMS:
Tablets: 5 mg

LINAGLIPTIN/
METFORMIN
LIN a GLIP tin/MET for MIN
TRADE NAME(S):
Jentadueto
THERAPEUTIC CLASS:
Antidiabetic
GENERAL USES:
Diabetes (type 2)
DOSAGE FORMS:
Tablets: 2.5 mg/500 mg,
2.5 mg/850 mg,
2.5 mg/1000 mg

LINDANE
LIN dane
TRADE NAME(S):
Kwell, G-well
THERAPEUTIC CLASS:
Scabicide/pediculicide
(topical)
GENERAL USES:
Scabies, head lice
DOSAGE FORMS:
Lotion and
Shampoo: 1%

LINEZOLID
li NE zoh lid
TRADE NAME(S):
Zyvox
THERAPEUTIC CLASS:
Anti-infective
GENERAL USES:
Vancomycin-resistant
bacterial infections
DOSAGE FORMS:
Tablets: 400 mg, 600 mg;
Suspension: 100 mg/
5 mL; Injection: 200 mg,
400 mg, 600 mg

LIOTHYRONINE
lye oh THYE roe neen
TRADE NAME(S):
Cytomel, Triostat
THERAPEUTIC CLASS:
Hormone (thyroid)
GENERAL USES:
Hypothyroidism

DOSAGE FORMS:
Tablets: 5 mcg, 25 mcg,
50 mcg; Injection: 10 mcg

LIRAGLUTIDE
LIR a GLOO tide
TRADE NAME(S):
Victoza
THERAPEUTIC CLASS:
Antidiabetic agent
GENERAL USES:
Diabetes (type 2)
DOSAGE FORMS:
Injection: 18 mg

LISDEXAMFETAMINE DIMESYLATE
lis DEX am FET a meen dye
MES i late
TRADE NAME(S):
Vyvanse
THERAPEUTIC CLASS:
Amphetamine
GENERAL USES:
ADHD
DOSAGE FORMS:
Capsules: 20 mg, 30 mg,
40 mg, 50 mg, 60 mg,
70 mg

LISINOPRIL
lyse IN oh pril
TRADE NAME(S):
Zestril, Prinivil
THERAPEUTIC CLASS:
Antihypertensive, cardiac
agent

GENERAL USES:
Hypertension, heart
failure, MI
DOSAGE FORMS:
Tablets: 2.5 mg, 5 mg,
10 mg, 20 mg, 40 mg

LISINOPRIL/HCTZ
lyse IN oh pril/hye droe klor
oh THYE a zide
TRADE NAME(S):
Zestoretic, Prinzide
THERAPEUTIC CLASS:
Antihypertensive/diuretic
GENERAL USES:
Hypertension
DOSAGE FORMS:
Tablets: 10 mg/12.5 mg,
20 mg/12.5 mg, 20 mg/
25 mg

LITHIUM
LITH ee um
TRADE NAME(S):
Eskalith, Eskalith CR,
Lithotabs, Lithobid
THERAPEUTIC CLASS:
Antipsychotic
GENERAL USES:
Psychotic disorders
DOSAGE FORMS:
Capsules: 150 mg,
300 mg, 600 mg; Tablets:
300 mg; Sustained-
release tablets: 300 mg;
Controlled-release tablets:
450 mg; Syrup: 8 mEq or
300 mg/5 mL

LODOXAMIDE
loe DOKS a mide
TRADE NAME(S):
Alomide
THERAPEUTIC CLASS:
Ocular agent
GENERAL USES:
Allergic conjunctivitis
DOSAGE FORMS:
Ophthalmic solution: 0.1%

LOMEFLOXACIN
loe me FLOKS a sin
TRADE NAME(S):
Maxaquin
THERAPEUTIC CLASS:
Anti-infective
GENERAL USES:
Bacterial infections
DOSAGE FORMS:
Tablets: 400 mg

LOMITAPIDE MESYLATE
loe MI ta pide
TRADE NAME(S):
Juxtapid
THERAPEUTIC CLASS:
Antilipemic
GENERAL USES:
Hyperlipidemia
DOSAGE FORMS:
Capsules: 5 mg, 10 mg,
20 mg

**LOPINAVIR/
RITONAVIR**
loe PIN a veer/ri TOE na veer
TRADE NAME(S):
Kaletra

THERAPEUTIC CLASS:
Antiviral
GENERAL USES:
HIV infection
DOSAGE FORMS:
Solution: 80 mg/20 mg
per mL; Tablets: 200 mg/
500 mg

LORATADINE
lor AT a deen
TRADE NAME(S):
Claritin
THERAPEUTIC CLASS:
Antihistamine
GENERAL USES:
Allergic rhinitis/hives
DOSAGE FORMS:
Tablets: 10 mg; Syrup:
1 mg/mL (240 mL);
Rapidly disintegrating
tablets: 10 mg

**LORATIDINE/
PSEUDOEPHEDRINE**
lor AT a deen/soo doe e
FED rin
TRADE NAME(S):
Claritin-D, Claritin-D
24 Hour
THERAPEUTIC CLASS:
Antihistamine/
decongestant
GENERAL USES:
Allergic rhinitis
DOSAGE FORMS:
Tablets: 5 mg/120 mg (D),
10 mg/240 mg (D-24)

LORAZEPAM
lor A ze pam
TRADE NAME(S):
Ativan
THERAPEUTIC CLASS:
Antianxiety agent
GENERAL USES:
Anxiety, sedation
DOSAGE FORMS:
Tablets: 0.5 mg, 1 mg,
2 mg; Concentrated
solution: 2 mg/mL;
Injection: 2 mg, 4 mg,
8 mg, 20 mg, 40 mg

LORCASERIN HCL
lor ca SER in
TRADE NAME(S):
Belviq
THERAPEUTIC CLASS:
Anorexiant
GENERAL USES:
Weight management
DOSAGE FORMS:
Tablets: 10 mg

LOSARTAN
loe SAR tan
TRADE NAME(S):
Cozaar
THERAPEUTIC CLASS:
Antihypertensive
GENERAL USES:
Hypertension, diabetic
nephropathy
DOSAGE FORMS:
Tablets: 25 mg, 50 mg,
100 mg

LOSARTAN/HCTZ
loe SAR tan/hye droe klor oh
THYE a zide
TRADE NAME(S):
Hyzaar
THERAPEUTIC CLASS:
Antihypertensive/diuretic
GENERAL USES:
Hypertension
DOSAGE FORMS:
Tablets: 50 mg/12.5 mg,
100 mg/25 mg

LOTEPREDNOL
loe te PRED nol
TRADE NAME(S):
Lotemax, Alrex
THERAPEUTIC CLASS:
Ocular agent
GENERAL USES:
Ocular inflammation,
allergies
DOSAGE FORMS:
Ophthalmic suspension:
0.2%, 0.5%; Ophthalmic
gel: 0.5%

**LOTEPREDNOL/
TOBRAMYCIN**
loe te PRED nol/toe bra MYE
sin
TRADE NAME(S):
Zylet
THERAPEUTIC CLASS:
Ocular agent
GENERAL USES:
Ocular inflammation/
infection

DOSAGE FORMS:
Ophthalmic solution:
0.5%/0.3%

LOVASTATIN
LOE va sta tin
TRADE NAME(S):
Mevacor, Altocor
THERAPEUTIC CLASS:
Antilipemic
GENERAL USES:
Hyperlipidemia,
atherosclerosis
DOSAGE FORMS:
Tablets: 10 mg, 20 mg,
40 mg; Extended-release
tablets: 10 mg, 20 mg,
40 mg, 60 mg

LOVASTATIN/NIACIN
LOE va sta tin/NYE a sin
TRADE NAME(S):
Advicor
THERAPEUTIC CLASS:
Antilipemic
GENERAL USES:
Hyperlipidemia
DOSAGE FORMS:
Caplets: 20 mg/1 g,
20 mg/750 mg, 20 mg/
500 mg

LOXAPINE
LOKS a peen
TRADE NAME(S):
Adasure, Loxitane,
Loxitane C

THERAPEUTIC CLASS:
Antipsychotic
GENERAL USES:
Psychotic disorders
DOSAGE FORMS:
Capsules: 5 mg,
10 mg, 25 mg, 50 mg;
Concentrated solution:
25 mg/mL; Injection:
500 mg; Inhalation: 10 mg

LUBIPROSTONE
loo bi PROS tone
TRADE NAME(S):
Amitiza
THERAPEUTIC CLASS:
Laxative
GENERAL USES:
Chronic idiopathic
constipation, opiod-
induced constipation
DOSAGE FORMS:
Capsules: 24 mcg

LUCINACTANT
LOO sin AK tant
TRADE NAME(S):
Surfaxin
THERAPEUTIC CLASS:
Respiratory agent
GENERAL USES:
RDS in premature infants
DOSAGE FORMS:
Suspension
(intratracheal): 8.5 mL

LULICONAZOLE
LOO li KON a zole
TRADE NAME(S):
Luzu
THERAPEUTIC CLASS:
Antifungal
GENERAL USES:
Athlete's foot, jock itch,
ringworm
DOSAGE FORMS:
Cream: 1%

LURASIDONE HCL
loo RAS i done
TRADE NAME(S):
Latuda
THERAPEUTIC CLASS:
Antipsychotic
GENERAL USES:
Schizophrenia, bipolar
depression
DOSAGE FORMS:
Tablets: 20 mg, 40 mg,
80 mg, 120 mg

MACITENTAN
MA si TEN tan
TRADE NAME(S):
Opsumit
THERAPEUTIC CLASS:
Cardiac agent
GENERAL USES:
Pulmonary hypertension
DOSAGE FORMS:
Tablets: 10 mg

MAGNESIUM SULFATE
mag NEE zhum
TRADE NAME(S):
Magnesium Sulfate
THERAPEUTIC CLASS:
Electrolyte
GENERAL USES:
Anticonvulsant,
replacement
DOSAGE FORMS:
Injection: 10%, 12.5%,
50%

**MANNITOL
(INHALATION)**
MAN i tole
TRADE NAME(S):
Aridol
THERAPEUTIC CLASS:
Diagnostic
GENERAL USES:
Diagnosis of bronchial
hyperresponsiveness
DOSAGE FORMS:
Inhalation: 5 mg, 10 mg,
20 mg, 40 mg

MAPROTILINE
ma PROE ti leen
TRADE NAME(S):
Ludiomil
THERAPEUTIC CLASS:
Antidepressant
GENERAL USES:
Depression
DOSAGE FORMS:
Tablets: 25 mg, 50 mg,
75 mg

MARAVIROC
mah RAV er rock
Trade Name(s):
Selzentry
Therapeutic Class:
Antiviral
General Uses:
HIV infection
Dosage Forms:
Tablets: 150 mg, 300 mg

**MECASERMIN
RINFABATE
(rDNA ORIGIN)**
mek a SER min
Trade Name(s):
Iplex
Therapeutic Class:
Hormone
General Uses:
Growth failure in children
Dosage Forms:
Injection: 36 mg

**MECASERMIN
(rDNA ORIGIN)**
mek a SER min
Trade Name(s):
Increlex
Therapeutic Class:
Hormone
General Uses:
Growth failure in children
Dosage Forms:
Injection: 40 mg

MECHLORETHAMINE
mech klor EH tha meen
Trade Name(s):
Valchlor
Therapeutic Class:
Antineoplastic
General Uses:
Cutaneous T-cell
lymphoma
Dosage Forms:
Gel: 0.016%

MECLIZINE
MEK li zeen
Trade Name(s):
Antivert, Antrizine, Vergon
Therapeutic Class:
Antiemetic/antivertigo
agent
General Uses:
Motion sickness
Dosage Forms:
Tablets: 12.5 mg, 25 mg,
50 mg; Capsules: 25 mg,
30 mg; Chewable tablets:
25 mg

**MEDROXY-
PROGESTERONE
ACETATE**
me DROKS ee proe JES te
rone
Trade Name(s):
Provera, Cycrin, Amen
Therapeutic Class:
Hormone (progestin)

GENERAL USES:
Amenorrhea, uterine
bleeding

DOSAGE FORMS:
Tablets: 2.5 mg, 5 mg,
10 mg

MEDROXY-PROGESTERONE ACETATE
me DROKS ee proe JES te
rone

TRADE NAME(S):
Depo-Provera, Depo-
SubQ Provera 104

THERAPEUTIC CLASS:
Hormone (progestin)

GENERAL USES:
Contraception

DOSAGE FORMS:
Injection: 150 mg, 104 mg

MEFENAMIC ACID
me fe NAM ik

TRADE NAME(S):
Ponstel

THERAPEUTIC CLASS:
Anti-inflammatory/
analgesic

GENERAL USES:
Menstrual cramping and
pain

DOSAGE FORMS:
Capsules: 250 mg

MEFLOQUINE
ME floe kwin

TRADE NAME(S):
Lariam

THERAPEUTIC CLASS:
Antimalarial

GENERAL USES:
Malaria treatment and
prevention

DOSAGE FORMS:
Tablets: 250 mg

MEGESTROL ACETATE
me JES trole

TRADE NAME(S):
Megace, Megace ES

THERAPEUTIC CLASS:
Hormone (progestin)

GENERAL USES:
Appetite enhancement,
breast/endometrium
cancers (palliative)

DOSAGE FORMS:
Tablets: 20 mg, 40 mg;
Suspension: 40 mg/mL;
Concentrate: 625 mg/
5 mL

MELOXICAM
mel OKS i kam

TRADE NAME(S):
Mobic

THERAPEUTIC CLASS:
Anti-inflammatory/
analgesic

GENERAL USES:
Osteoarthritis, rheumatoid
arthritis

DOSAGE FORMS:
Tablets: 7.5 mg;
Suspension: 7.5 mg/5 mL

MEMANTINE
me MAN teen
TRADE NAME(S):
Namenda, Namenda XR
THERAPEUTIC CLASS:
Alzheimer's agent
GENERAL USES:
Alzheimer's disease
DOSAGE FORMS:
Extended-release
capsules: 7 mg, 14 mg,
21 mg, 28 mg; Tablets:
5 mg, 10 mg;
Solution: 2 mg/mL

MEPERIDINE
me PER i deen
TRADE NAME(S):
Demerol
THERAPEUTIC CLASS:
Analgesic (narcotic)
GENERAL USES:
Pain
DOSAGE FORMS:
Tablets: 50 mg, 100 mg;
Syrup: 50 mg/5 mL;
Injection: 25 mg, 50 mg,
75 mg, 100 mg

MEQUINOL/TRETINOIN
ME kwi nole/TRET i noyn
TRADE NAME(S):
Solage
THERAPEUTIC CLASS:
Skin agent (topical)
GENERAL USES:
Aging solar skin spots

DOSAGE FORMS:
Solution: 2%/0.01%

MERCAPTOPURINE
mer KAP toe PURE een
TRADE NAME(S):
Purinethol, Purixan
THERAPEUTIC CLASS:
Antineoplastic
GENERAL USES:
ALL
DOSAGE FORMS:
Tablets: 50 mg;
Suspension: 20 mg/mL

MEROPENEM
mer oh PEN em
TRADE NAME(S):
Merrem IV
THERAPEUTIC CLASS:
Anti-infective
GENERAL USES:
Bacterial infections
DOSAGE FORMS:
Injection: 500 mg, 1 g

MESALAMINE
me SAL a meen
TRADE NAME(S):
Apriso, Asacol, Lialda,
Pentasa, Rowasa Rectal,
Delzicol
THERAPEUTIC CLASS:
GI agent
GENERAL USES:
Inflammatory bowel
disease

DOSAGE FORMS:
Delayed-release tablets: 400 mg, 1.2 g; Controlled-release capsules: 250 mg; Delayed-release capsules: 40 mg; Extended-release capsules: 375 mg; Rectal enema: 4 g/60 mL; Suppository (rectal): 500 mg

MESORIDAZINE
mez oh RID a zeen
TRADE NAME(S):
Serentil
THERAPEUTIC CLASS:
Antipsychotic
GENERAL USES:
Psychotic disorders
DOSAGE FORMS:
Tablets: 10 mg, 25 mg, 50 mg, 100 mg; Concentrated solution: 25 mg/mL; Injection: 25 mg

MESTRANOL/ NORETHINDRONE
MES tra nole/nor eth IN drone
TRADE NAME(S):
Genora 1/50, Nelova 1/50M, Norethin 1/50M, Norinyl 1+50, Necon 1/50, Ortho-Novum 1/50

THERAPEUTIC CLASS:
Contraceptive (monophasic)
GENERAL USES:
Contraception
DOSAGE FORMS:
Tablets: 50 mcg/1 mg

METAPROTERENOL
met a proe TER e nol
TRADE NAME(S):
Alupent
THERAPEUTIC CLASS:
Bronchodilator
GENERAL USES:
Bronchospasm, asthma
DOSAGE FORMS:
Tablets: 10 mg, 20 mg; Syrup: 10 mg/5 mL; Aerosol: 5 mL, 10 mL; Inhalation solution: 0.4%, 0.6%, 5%

METAXALONE
me TAKS a lone
TRADE NAME(S):
Skelaxin
THERAPEUTIC CLASS:
Skeletal muscle relaxant
GENERAL USES:
Musculoskeletal conditions
DOSAGE FORMS:
Tablets: 800 mg

METFORMIN
met FOR min

Trade Name(s):
Fortamet, Glucophage,
Glucophage XR, Glumetza

Therapeutic Class:
Antidiabetic

General Uses:
Diabetes (type 2)

Dosage Forms:
Tablets: 500 mg, 850 mg,
1000 mg; Extended-
release tablets: 100 mg,
500 mg, 750 mg, 1000 mg

METFORMIN/
GLIPIZIDE
met FOR min/GLIP i zide

Trade Name(s):
Metaglip

Therapeutic Class:
Antidiabetic

General Uses:
Diabetes

Dosage Forms:
Tablets: 250 mg/2.5 mg,
500 mg/2.5 mg, 500 mg/
5 mg

METFORMIN/
PIOGLITAZONE
met FOR min/pye oh GLI ta
zone

Trade Name(s):
Actoplus Met, Actoplus
Met XR

Therapeutic Class:
Antidiabetic

General Uses:
Diabetes

Dosage Forms:
Tablets: 500 mg/15 mg,
850 mg/15 mg;
Extended-release tablets:
1000 mg/15 mg,
1000 mg/30 mg

METFORMIN/
SAXAGLIPTIN
met FOR min/SAX a GLIP tin

Trade Name(s):
Kombiglyze XR

Therapeutic Class:
Antidiabetic

General Uses:
Diabetes (type 2)

Dosage Forms:
Extended-release tablets:
500 mg/5 mg, 1000 mg/
5 mg, 1000 mg/2.5 mg

METHIMAZOLE
meth IM a zole

Trade Name(s):
Tapazole

Therapeutic Class:
Antithyroid agent

General Uses:
Hyperthyroidism

Dosage Forms:
Tablets: 5 mg, 10 mg

METHOCARBAMOL
meth oh KAR ba mole

Trade Name(s):
Robaxin

THERAPEUTIC CLASS:
  Skeletal muscle
  relaxant
GENERAL USES:
  Musculoskeletal
  conditions
DOSAGE FORMS:
  Tablets: 500 mg, 750 mg

METHOTREXATE
meth oh TREKS ate
TRADE NAME(S):
  Otrexup, Raguro,
  Rheumatrex, Trexall
THERAPEUTIC CLASS:
  Antineoplastic,
  antirheumatic
GENERAL USES:
  Cancer, rheumatoid
  arthritis, psoriasis
DOSAGE FORMS:
  Tablets: 2.5 mg, 5 mg,
  7.5 mg, 10 mg, 15 mg;
  Injection: 7.5 mg, 10 mg,
  12.5 mg, 15 mg, 17.5 mg,
  20 mg, 22.5 mg, 25 mg,
  27.5 mg, 30 mg, 50 mg,
  250 mg, 1 g

METHOXY POLYETHYLENE GLYCOL EPOETIN BETA
meth OKS ee pol ee ETH
i leen GLY kol e POE e tin
BAY ta
TRADE NAME(S):
  Mircera

THERAPEUTIC CLASS:
  Hematological agent
GENERAL USES:
  Anemia
DOSAGE FORMS:
  Injection: 50 mcg,
  75 mcg, 100 mcg,
  150 mcg, 200 mcg,
  250 mcg, 300 mcg,
  400 mcg, 600 mcg,
  800 mcg, 1000 mcg

METHYLDOPA
meth il DOE pa
TRADE NAME(S):
  Aldomet
THERAPEUTIC CLASS:
  Antihypertensive
GENERAL USES:
  Hypertension
DOSAGE FORMS:
  Tablets: 125 mg, 250 mg,
  500 mg; Suspension:
  250 mg/5 mL; Injection:
  250 mg (methyldopate)

METHYLDOPA/HCTZ
meth il DOE pa/hye droe klor
oh THYE a zide
TRADE NAME(S):
  Aldoril
THERAPEUTIC CLASS:
  Antihypertensive/
  diuretic
GENERAL USES:
  Hypertension
DOSAGE FORMS:
  Tablets: 250 mg/15 mg,

250 mg/25 mg, 500 mg/
30 mg, 500 mg/50 mg

METHYLNALTREXONE
meth il nal TREKS one
TRADE NAME(S):
Relistor
THERAPEUTIC CLASS:
GI agent
GENERAL USES:
Opioid-induced
constipation
DOSAGE FORMS:
Injection: 12 mg

METHYLPHENIDATE
meth il FEN i date
TRADE NAME(S):
Concerta, Metadate,
Metadate CD, Ritalin,
Ritalin LA, Methylin,
Quillivant XR
THERAPEUTIC CLASS:
CNS stimulant
GENERAL USES:
ADHD, narcolepsy
DOSAGE FORMS:
Tablets: 5 mg, 10 mg,
20 mg; Sustained-release
tablets or capsules:
20 mg; Extended-release
tablets: 10 mg, 18 mg,
20 mg, 27 mg, 36 mg,
54 mg; Extended-release
capsules: 10 mg, 20 mg,
30 mg, 40 mg;
Oral solution: 5 mg/5 mL,

10 mg/5 mL; Extended-
release oral suspension:
25 mg/5 mL; Chewable
tablets: 2.5 mg, 5 mg,
10 mg

METHYLPHENIDATE
(TRANSDERMAL)
meth il FEN i date
TRADE NAME(S):
Daytrana
THERAPEUTIC CLASS:
CNS stimulant
GENERAL USES:
ADHD (age 6 to 12 yr)
DOSAGE FORMS:
Patch: 15 mg

METHYLPREDNISOLONE
meth il pred NIS oh lone
TRADE NAME(S):
Medrol
THERAPEUTIC CLASS:
Glucocorticoid
GENERAL USES:
Endocrine, skin, blood
disorders
DOSAGE FORMS:
Tablets: 2 mg, 4 mg,
8 mg, 16 mg, 24 mg,
32 mg

METHYLPREDNISOLONE
ACETATE
meth il pred NIS oh lone
TRADE NAME(S):
Depo-Medrol, Depoject,
Depopred

Therapeutic Class:
Glucocorticoid

General Uses:
Endocrine, skin, blood disorders

Dosage Forms:
Injection: 40 mg, 80 mg, 100 mg, 200 mg, 400 mg

METHYLPREDNISOLONE SODIUM SUCCINATE
meth il pred NIS oh lone

Trade Name(s):
A-Methapred, Solu-Medrol

Therapeutic Class:
Glucocorticoid

General Uses:
Endocrine, skin, blood disorders

Dosage Forms:
Injection: 40 mg, 125 mg, 500 mg, 1 g, 2 g

METHYSERGIDE
meth i SER jide

Trade Name(s):
Sansert

Therapeutic Class:
Antimigraine agent

General Uses:
Migraines

Dosage Forms:
Tablets: 2 mg

METIPRANOLOL
met i PRAN oh lol

Trade Name(s):
OptiPranolol

Therapeutic Class:
Ocular agent

General Uses:
Glaucoma/ocular hypertension

Dosage Forms:
Ophthalmic solution: 0.3%

METOCLOPRAMIDE
met oh KLOE pra mide

Trade Name(s):
Reglan, Clopra, Maxolon, Metozolv ODT, Octamide, Reclomide

Therapeutic Class:
Antiemetic

General Uses:
Nausea, vomiting

Dosage Forms:
Orally disintegrating tablets and Tablets: 5 mg, 10 mg; Syrup: 5 mg/5 mL; Concentrated solution: 10 mg/mL; Injection: 10 mg, 50 mg, 150 mg

METOLAZONE
me TOLE a zone

Trade Name(s):
Mykrox, Zaroxolyn

Therapeutic Class:
Diuretic

GENERAL USES:
CHF-related edema,
hypertension
DOSAGE FORMS:
Tablets: 0.5 mg, 2.5 mg,
5 mg, 10 mg

METOPROLOL
me toe PROE lole
TRADE NAME(S):
Lopressor, Toprol-XL
THERAPEUTIC CLASS:
Antihypertensive,
antianginal, cardiac agent
GENERAL USES:
Hypertension, angina, MI
DOSAGE FORMS:
Tablets: 25 mg, 50 mg,
100 mg; Extended-release
tablets: 25 mg, 50 mg,
100 mg, 200 mg;
Injection: 5 mg

METOPROLOL/HCTZ
me toe PROE lole/hye dro
klor oh THYE a zide
TRADE NAME(S):
Lopressor HCT
THERAPEUTIC CLASS:
Antihypertensive/
diuretic
GENERAL USES:
Hypertension
DOSAGE FORMS:
Tablets: 50 mg/25 mg,
100 mg/25 mg, 100 mg/
50 mg

METRELEPTIN
MET re LEP tin
TRADE NAME(S):
Myalept
THERAPEUTIC CLASS:
Leptin analog
GENERAL USES:
Leptin deficiency
DOSAGE FORMS:
Injection: 11.3 mg

METRONIDAZOLE
me troe NI da zole
TRADE NAME(S):
Flagyl, Flagyl IV
THERAPEUTIC CLASS:
Anti-infective
GENERAL USES:
Bacterial infections,
gastric ulcers
DOSAGE FORMS:
Tablets: 250 mg, 500 mg;
Extended-release tablets:
750 mg; Capsules:
375 mg; Injection: 500 mg

METRONIDAZOLE
(TOPICAL)
me troe NI da zole
TRADE NAME(S):
MetroGel, MetroLotion,
Noritate
THERAPEUTIC CLASS:
Anti-infective (topical)
GENERAL USES:
Rosacea acne

DOSAGE FORMS:
Gel and Lotion: 0.75%;
Cream: 1%

METRONIDAZOLE (VAGINAL)
me troe NI da zole
TRADE NAME(S):
MetroGel-Vaginal
THERAPEUTIC CLASS:
Vaginal anti-infective
GENERAL USES:
Bacterial vaginosis
DOSAGE FORMS:
Gel: 0.75%, 1.3%

MEXILETINE
meks IL e teen
TRADE NAME(S):
Mexitil
THERAPEUTIC CLASS:
Antiarrhythmic
GENERAL USES:
Arrhythmias,
tachycardia
DOSAGE FORMS:
Capsules: 150 mg,
200 mg, 250 mg

MEZLOCILLIN
mez loe SIL in
TRADE NAME(S):
Mezlin
THERAPEUTIC CLASS:
Anti-infective
GENERAL USES:
Bacterial infections

DOSAGE FORMS:
Injection: 1 g, 2 g, 3 g,
4 g, 20 g

MICAFUNGIN SODIUM
mi ka FUN gin
TRADE NAME(S):
Mycamine
THERAPEUTIC CLASS:
Antifungal
GENERAL USES:
Candida infections
DOSAGE FORMS:
Injection: 50 mg

MICONAZOLE (BUCCAL)
mi KON a zole
TRADE NAME(S):
Oravig
THERAPEUTIC CLASS:
Antifungal
GENERAL USES:
Oral candidiasis
DOSAGE FORMS:
Buccal tablets: 50 mg

MICONAZOLE (VAGINAL)
mi KON a zole
TRADE NAME(S):
Monistat-3, Monistat-
Derm
THERAPEUTIC CLASS:
Vaginal antifungal
GENERAL USES:
Vaginal candidiasis
DOSAGE FORMS:
Vaginal suppository:
200 mg; Topical cream:
2%

MICONAZOLE/ZINC OXIDE/WHITE PETROLATUM

mi KON a zole

TRADE NAME(S):
Vusion

THERAPEUTIC CLASS:
Dermatological agent

GENERAL USES:
Diaper dermatitis/
candidiasis

DOSAGE FORMS:
Ointment: 30 g

MIDAZOLAM

mi DAZ oh lam

TRADE NAME(S):
Versed

THERAPEUTIC CLASS:
Sedative

GENERAL USES:
Pre-op sedation

DOSAGE FORMS:
Syrup: 2 mg/mL;
Injection: 2 mg, 5 mg,
10 mg, 25 mg, 50 mg

MIFEPRISTONE

mi FE pris tone

TRADE NAME(S):
Mifeprex

THERAPEUTIC CLASS:
Progesterone
antagonist

GENERAL USES:
Abortifacient

DOSAGE FORMS:
Tablets: 200 mg

MIFEPRISTONE

mi FE pris tone

TRADE NAME(S):
Korlym

THERAPEUTIC CLASS:
Antidiabetic

GENERAL USES:
Diabetes (type 2), high
glucose levels related to
Cushing's syndrome

DOSAGE FORMS:
Tablets: 300 mg

MIGLITOL

MIG li tol

TRADE NAME(S):
Glyset

THERAPEUTIC CLASS:
Antidiabetic

GENERAL USES:
Diabetes (type 2)

DOSAGE FORMS:
Tablets: 25 mg, 50 mg,
100 mg

MIGLUSTAT

MIG loo stat

TRADE NAME(S):
Zavesca

THERAPEUTIC CLASS:
Enzyme inhibitor

GENERAL USES:
Gaucher's disease

DOSAGE FORMS:
Capsules: 100 mg

MILNACIPRAN HCL
mil NA si pran
TRADE NAME(S):
  Savella
THERAPEUTIC CLASS:
  Miscellaneous
GENERAL USES:
  Fibromyalgia
DOSAGE FORMS:
  Tablets: 12.5 mg, 25 mg,
  50 mg, 100 mg

MILTEFOSINE
MIL te FOE seen
TRADE NAME(S):
  Impavido
THERAPEUTIC CLASS:
  Antiparasitic
GENERAL USES:
  Leishmaniasis
DOSAGE FORMS:
  Capsules: 50 mg

MINOCYCLINE
mi noe SYE kleen
TRADE NAME(S):
  Dynacin, Vectrin, Minocin,
  Solodyn, Ximino
THERAPEUTIC CLASS:
  Anti-infective
GENERAL USES:
  Bacterial infections, acne
DOSAGE FORMS:
  Tablets and Capsules:
  50 mg, 75 mg, 100 mg;
  Extended-release
  capsules: 67.5 mg,
  112.5 mg; Extended-
  release capsules and
  tablets: 45 mg, 90 mg,
  135 mg; Suspension:
  50 mg/5 mL

MINOXIDIL
mi NOKS i dil
TRADE NAME(S):
  Loniten
THERAPEUTIC CLASS:
  Antihypertensive
GENERAL USES:
  Hypertension
DOSAGE FORMS:
  Tablets: 2.5 mg, 10 mg

MIPOMERSEN SODIUM
MYE poe mer sen
TRADE NAME(S):
  Kynamro
THERAPEUTIC CLASS:
  Antilipemic
GENERAL USES:
  Hyperlipidemia
DOSAGE FORMS:
  Injection: 200 mg

MIRABEGRON
MIR a BEG ron
TRADE NAME(S):
  Myrbetriq
THERAPEUTIC CLASS:
  Anticholinergic
GENERAL USES:
  Overactive bladder

Dosage Forms:
   Extended-release tablets:
   25 mg, 50 mg

MIRTAZAPINE
mir TAZ a peen
Trade Name(s):
   Remeron
Therapeutic Class:
   Antidepressant
General Uses:
   Depression
Dosage Forms:
   Tablets and Orally
   disintegrating tablets:
   7.5 mg (orally
   disintegrating only),
   15 mg, 30 mg, 45 mg

MISOPROSTOL
mye soe PROST ole
Trade Name(s):
   Cytotec
Therapeutic Class:
   Gastric protectant
General Uses:
   Prevention of NSAID
   gastric ulcer
Dosage Forms:
   Tablets: 100 mcg,
   200 mcg

MODAFINIL
moe DAF i nil
Trade Name(s):
   Provigil
Therapeutic Class:
   CNS stimulant

General Uses:
   Narcolepsy, improve
   fatigue associated with
   sleep apnea and sleep
   disorders
Dosage Forms:
   Tablets: 100 mg, 200 mg

MOEXIPRIL
mo EKS i pril
Trade Name(s):
   Univasc
Therapeutic Class:
   Antihypertensive, cardiac
   agent
General Uses:
   Hypertension, left
   ventricular dysfunction
Dosage Forms:
   Tablets: 7.5 mg, 15 mg

MOEXIPRIL/HCTZ
mo EKS i pril/hye droe klor
oh THYE a zide
Trade Name(s):
   Uniretic
Therapeutic Class:
   Antihypertensive/
   diuretic
General Uses:
   Hypertension
Dosage Forms:
   Tablets: 15 mg/25 mg,
   7.5 mg/12.5 mg

MOLINDONE
moe LIN done
TRADE NAME(S):
Moban
THERAPEUTIC CLASS:
Antipsychotic
GENERAL USES:
Psychotic disorders
DOSAGE FORMS:
Tablets: 5 mg, 10 mg,
25 mg, 50 mg

MOMETASONE (NASAL)
moe MET a sone
TRADE NAME(S):
Nasonex
THERAPEUTIC CLASS:
Corticosteroid (nasal)
GENERAL USES:
Allergies
DOSAGE FORMS:
Nasal spray: 50 mcg/
spray

MOMETASONE (TOPICAL)
moe MET a sone
TRADE NAME(S):
Elocon
THERAPEUTIC CLASS:
Corticosteroid (topical)
GENERAL USES:
Various skin
conditions
DOSAGE FORMS:
Ointment, Cream, and
Lotion: 0.1%

MOMETASONE FUROATE (ORAL INHALER)
moe MET a sone
FYOOR oh ate
TRADE NAME(S):
Asmanex, Asmanex HFA
THERAPEUTIC CLASS:
Corticosteroid
GENERAL USES:
Asthma
DOSAGE FORMS:
Oral inhalation: 100 mcg/
inhalation, 200 mcg/
inhalation, 220 mcg/
inhalation

MONTELUKAST
mon te LOO kast
TRADE NAME(S):
Singulair
THERAPEUTIC CLASS:
Bronchodilator
GENERAL USES:
Asthma prevention and
treatment, seasonal
allergies
DOSAGE FORMS:
Tablets: 10 mg;
Chewable tablets:
4 mg, 5 mg;
Granules: 4 mg

MORICIZINE
mor I siz een
TRADE NAME(S):
Ethmozine
THERAPEUTIC CLASS:
Antiarrhythmic

GENERAL USES:
Arrhythmias
DOSAGE FORMS:
Tablets: 200 mg, 250 mg, 300 mg

MORPHINE SULFATE
MOR feen
TRADE NAME(S):
Avinza, MS Contin, Oramorph SR, Kadian, Roxanol, Duramorph, Infumorph
THERAPEUTIC CLASS:
Analgesic (narcotic)
GENERAL USES:
Pain
DOSAGE FORMS:
Tablets: 15 mg, 30 mg; Controlled-release tablets: 15 mg, 30 mg, 60 mg, 100 mg, 200 mg; Soluble tablets: 10 mg, 15 mg, 30 mg; Capsules: 15 mg, 30 mg; Sustained-release capsules: 20 mg, 50 mg, 100 mg; Extended-release capsules: 30 mg, 60 mg, 90 mg, 120 mg; Solution: various concentrations; Injection: various concentrations

MORPHINE SULFATE (LIPOSOMAL)
MOR feen
TRADE NAME(S):
DepoDur

THERAPEUTIC CLASS:
Analgesic (narcotic)
GENERAL USES:
Major pain following surgery (single-dose administration)
DOSAGE FORMS:
Injection: 10 mg, 15 mg, 20 mg

MORPHINE SULFATE/ NALTREXONE
MOR feen SUL fate/ nal TREKS one
TRADE NAME(S):
Embeda
THERAPEUTIC CLASS:
Analgesic (narcotic)
GENERAL USES:
Pain
DOSAGE FORMS:
Extended-release capsules: 20 mg/0.8 mg, 30 mg/1.2 mg, 50 mg/ 2 mg, 60 mg/2.4 mg, 80 mg/3.2 mg, 100 mg/ 4 mg

MOXIFLOXACIN
moks i FLOKS a sin
TRADE NAME(S):
Avelox
THERAPEUTIC CLASS:
Anti-infective
GENERAL USES:
Bacterial infections

DOSAGE FORMS:
Tablets: 400 mg;
Injection: 400 mg

**MOXIFLOXACIN
(OCULAR)**
moks i FLOKS a sin
TRADE NAME(S):
Vigamox
THERAPEUTIC CLASS:
Ocular agent
(anti-infective)
GENERAL USES:
Bacterial
conjunctivitis
DOSAGE FORMS:
Ophthalmic solution:
0.5%

MUPIROCIN
myoo PEER oh sin
TRADE NAME(S):
Bactroban
THERAPEUTIC CLASS:
Anti-infective (topical)
GENERAL USES:
Impetigo, skin infections
DOSAGE FORMS:
Ointment and Cream: 2%

**MYCOPHENOLATE
MOFETIL**
mye koe FEN oh late MOE
feh till
TRADE NAME(S):
CellCept
THERAPEUTIC CLASS:
Immunosuppressant

GENERAL USES:
Prevent organ transplant
rejection
DOSAGE FORMS:
Capsules: 250 mg;
Tablets: 180 mg, 360 mg,
500 mg; Suspension:
200 mg/mL

NABILONE
NA bi lone
TRADE NAME(S):
Cesamet
THERAPEUTIC CLASS:
Antiemetic
GENERAL USES:
Chemotherapy-related
nausea and vomiting
DOSAGE FORMS:
Capsules: 1 mg

NABUMETONE
na BYOO me tone
TRADE NAME(S):
Relafen
THERAPEUTIC CLASS:
Anti-inflammatory/
analgesic
GENERAL USES:
Osteoarthritis, rheumatoid
arthritis
DOSAGE FORMS:
Tablets: 500 mg, 750 mg

NADOLOL
nay DOE lole
TRADE NAME(S):
Corgard

THERAPEUTIC CLASS:
Antihypertensive,
antianginal
GENERAL USES:
Hypertension, angina
DOSAGE FORMS:
Tablets: 20 mg, 40 mg,
80 mg, 120 mg,
160 mg

NAFCILLIN
naf SIL in
TRADE NAME(S):
Unipen, Nallpen
THERAPEUTIC CLASS:
Anti-infective
GENERAL USES:
Bacterial infections
DOSAGE FORMS:
Capsules: 250 mg;
Injection: 500 mg, 1 g,
2 g, 10 g

NAFTIFINE
NAF ti feen
TRADE NAME(S):
Naftin
THERAPEUTIC CLASS:
Antifungal (topical)
GENERAL USES:
Athlete's foot, jock itch,
ringworm
DOSAGE FORMS:
Cream: 1%; Gel: 1%, 2%

NALOXEGOL
nal OKS ee GOL
TRADE NAME(S):
Movantik
THERAPEUTIC CLASS:
GI agent
GENERAL CLASS:
Opioid-induced
constipation
DOSAGE FORMS:
Tablets: 12.5 mg, 25 mg

NALOXONE
nal OKS one
TRADE NAME(S):
Narcan, Evzio
THERAPEUTIC CLASS:
Antidote
GENERAL USES:
Reversal of opioid effects
DOSAGE FORMS:
Injection: 0.04 mg,
0.4 mg, 0.8 mg, 2 mg,
4 mg, 10 mg

NALTREXONE
nal TREKS one
TRADE NAME(S):
Depade, ReVia, Vivitrol
THERAPEUTIC CLASS:
Narcotic antagonist
GENERAL USES:
Treatment of alcohol
and opioid dependence;
blocks narcotic effects
DOSAGE FORMS:
Tablets: 25 mg, 50 mg,

100 mg; Injection
(extended release):
380 mg

NAPHAZOLINE
naf AZ oh leen
TRADE NAME(S):
  AK-Con, Albalon,
  Vasocon
THERAPEUTIC CLASS:
  Ocular agent
GENERAL USES:
  Ocular irritation
DOSAGE FORMS:
  Ophthalmic solution: 0.1%

NAPROXEN
na PROKS en
TRADE NAME(S):
  Anaprox DS, Aleve,
  Naprelan
THERAPEUTIC CLASS:
  Anti-inflammatory/
  analgesic
GENERAL USES:
  Osteoarthritis, rheumatoid
  arthritis, pain
DOSAGE FORMS:
  Tablets: 200 mg, 250 mg,
  375 mg, 500 mg;
  Delayed-release or
  Controlled-release
  tablets: 375 mg, 500 mg;
  Suspension: 125 mg/
  5 mL

NARATRIPTAN
NAR a trip tan
TRADE NAME(S):
  Amerge
THERAPEUTIC CLASS:
  Antimigraine agent
GENERAL USES:
  Migraines
DOSAGE FORMS:
  Tablets: 1 mg, 2.5 mg

NATALIZUMAB
nay tal IZ oo mab
TRADE NAME(S):
  Tysabri
THERAPEUTIC CLASS:
  Monoclonal antibody
GENERAL USES:
  Multiple sclerosis
DOSAGE FORMS:
  Injection: 300 mg

NATEGLINIDE
na te GLYE nide
TRADE NAME(S):
  Starlix
THERAPEUTIC CLASS:
  Antidiabetic
GENERAL USES:
  Diabetes (type 2)
DOSAGE FORMS:
  Tablets: 60 mg,
  120 mg

NEBIVOLOL
ne BIV oh lol
TRADE NAME(S):
  Bystolic

Therapeutic Class:
Antihypertensive
General Uses:
Hypertension
Dosage Forms:
Tablets: 2.5 mg, 5 mg,
10 mg

NEDOCROMIL
ne doe KROE mil
Trade Name(s):
Tilade
Therapeutic Class:
Respiratory inhalant
General Uses:
Asthma
Dosage Forms:
Inhaler: 1.75 mg/
inhalation

NEFAZODONE
nef AY zoe done
Trade Name(s):
Serzone
Therapeutic Class:
Antidepressant
General Uses:
Depression
Dosage Forms:
Tablets: 50 mg, 100 mg,
150 mg, 200 mg, 250 mg

NELARABINE
nel AY ra been
Trade Name(s):
Arranon
Therapeutic Class:
Antineoplastic

General Uses:
Lymphoblastic lymphoma,
leukemia
Dosage Forms:
Injection: 250 mg

NELFINAVIR
nel FIN a veer
Trade Name(s):
Viracept
Therapeutic Class:
Antiviral
General Uses:
HIV infection
Dosage Forms:
Tablets: 250 mg, 625 mg;
Powder: 50 mg/g

**NEOSTIGMINE
METHYLSULFATE**
nee o STIG meen meth IL
SUL fate
Trade Name(s):
Bloxiverz
Therapeutic Class:
Central nervous system
agent
General Uses:
Reversal of neuromuscular
blockade after surgery
Dosage Forms:
Injection: 5 mg, 10 mg

NEPAFENAC
ne pa FEN ak
Trade Name(s):
Nevanac, Ilevro

THERAPEUTIC CLASS:
Ocular agent
GENERAL USES:
Pain and inflammation after cataract surgery
DOSAGE FORMS:
Ophthalmic suspension: 0.1%, 0.3%

NESIRITIDE CITRATE
ni SIR i tide
TRADE NAME(S):
Natrecor
THERAPEUTIC CLASS:
Cardiac agent
GENERAL USES:
CHF
DOSAGE FORMS:
Injection: 1.5 mg

NETUPITANT/ PALONOSETRON
net YOO pit ant/PAL oh NOE se tron
TRADE NAME(S):
Akynzeo
THERAPEUTIC CLASS:
Antiemetic
GENERAL CLASS:
Chemotherapy-induced nausea/vomiting
DOSAGE FORMS:
Capsules: 300 mg/0.5 mg

NEVIRAPINE
ne VYE ra peen
TRADE NAME(S):
Viramune

THERAPEUTIC CLASS:
Antiviral
GENERAL USES:
HIV infection
DOSAGE FORMS:
Tablets: 200 mg; Suspension: 50 mg/5 mL

NIACIN (NICOTINIC ACID)
NYE a sin
TRADE NAME(S):
Niaspan
THERAPEUTIC CLASS:
Antilipemic
GENERAL USES:
Hyperlipidemia
DOSAGE FORMS:
Extended-release tablets: 500 mg, 750 mg, 1000 mg

NICARDIPINE
nye KAR de peen
TRADE NAME(S):
Cardene, Cardene SR, Cardene IV
THERAPEUTIC CLASS:
Antihypertensive, antianginal
GENERAL USES:
Hypertension, angina
DOSAGE FORMS:
Capsules: 20 mg, 30 mg; Sustained-release capsules: 30 mg, 45 mg, 60 mg; Injection: 25 mg

NIFEDIPINE
nye FED i peen
TRADE NAME(S):
Adalat, Procardia, Adalat CC, Procardia XL
THERAPEUTIC CLASS:
Antihypertensive (sustained release), antianginal
GENERAL USES:
Hypertension, angina
DOSAGE FORMS:
Capsules: 10 mg, 20 mg; Extended-release tablets: 30 mg, 60 mg, 90 mg

NILOTINIB
nye LOE ti nib
TRADE NAME(S):
Tasigna
THERAPEUTIC CLASS:
Antineoplastic
GENERAL USES:
Leukemia
DOSAGE FORMS:
Capsules: 200 mg

NILUTAMIDE
ni LOO ta mide
TRADE NAME(S):
Nilandron
THERAPEUTIC CLASS:
Antiandrogen/ antineoplastic
GENERAL USES:
Prostate cancer
DOSAGE FORMS:
Tablets: 50 mg

NIMODIPINE
nye MOE di peen
TRADE NAME(S):
Nimotop, Nymalize
THERAPEUTIC CLASS:
Cardiac agent
GENERAL USES:
Brain hemorrhage
DOSAGE FORMS:
Capsules: 30 mg; Solution: 60 mg/20 mL

NISOLDIPINE
nye SOL di peen
TRADE NAME(S):
Sular
THERAPEUTIC CLASS:
Antihypertensive
GENERAL USES:
Hypertension
DOSAGE FORMS:
Extended-release tablets: 10 mg, 20 mg, 30 mg, 40 mg

NITAZOXANIDE
nye ta ZOKS a nide
TRADE NAME(S):
Alinia
THERAPEUTIC CLASS:
Anti-infective
GENERAL USES:
Infectious diarrhea
DOSAGE FORMS:
Suspension: 100 mg/ 5 mL

NITROFURANTOIN
nye troe fyoor AN toyn

TRADE NAME(S):
Furadantin, Macrobid,
Macrodantin

THERAPEUTIC CLASS:
Anti-infective

GENERAL USES:
Urinary tract infections

DOSAGE FORMS:
Capsules: 25 mg, 50 mg,
100 mg; Oral suspension:
25 mg/5 mL

NITROGLYCERIN (INJECTION)
nye troe GLI ser in

TRADE NAME(S):
Tridil, Nitro-Bid IV

THERAPEUTIC CLASS:
Antianginal

GENERAL USES:
Angina

DOSAGE FORMS:
Injection: 5 mg, 25 mg,
50 mg, 100 mg

NITROGLYCERIN (RECTAL)
nye troe GLI ser in

TRADE NAME(S):
Rectiv

THERAPEUTIC CLASS:
Vasodilator

GENERAL USES:
Chronic anal fissure

DOSAGE FORMS:
Ointment (rectal): 0.4%

NITROGLYCERIN (SUBLINGUAL)
nye troe GLI ser in

TRADE NAME(S):
NitroQuick, Nitrostat,
Nitrolingual, Nitrotab

THERAPEUTIC CLASS:
Antianginal

GENERAL USES:
Angina

DOSAGE FORMS:
Sublingual tablets:
0.3 mg, 0.4 mg,
0.6 mg; Spray: 0.4 mg/
spray

NITROGLYCERIN (SUSTAINED RELEASE)
nye troe GLI ser in

TRADE NAME(S):
Nitrong, Nitroglyn, Nitro-
Time

THERAPEUTIC CLASS:
Antianginal

GENERAL USES:
Angina

DOSAGE FORMS:
Sustained-release
tablets: 2.6 mg, 6.5 mg,
9 mg; Sustained-release
capsules: 2.5 mg, 6.5 mg,
9 mg, 13 mg

NITROGLYCERIN (TOPICAL)
nye troe GLI ser in

TRADE NAME(S):
Nitrol, Nitro-Bid

THERAPEUTIC CLASS:
Antianginal (topical)
GENERAL USES:
Angina
DOSAGE FORMS:
Ointment: 2%

NITROGLYCERIN (TRANSDERMAL)
nye troe GLI ser in
TRADE NAME(S):
Minitran, Nitro-Dur,
Transderm-Nitro, Deponit
THERAPEUTIC CLASS:
Antianginal
GENERAL USES:
Angina
DOSAGE FORMS:
Release rate (mg/hr):
0.1 mg, 0.2 mg, 0.3 mg,
0.4 mg, 0.6 mg,
0.8 mg

NITROGLYCERIN (TRANSMUCOSAL-BUCCAL)
nye troe GLI ser in
TRADE NAME(S):
Nitrogard
THERAPEUTIC CLASS:
Antianginal
GENERAL USES:
Angina
DOSAGE FORMS:
Controlled-release tablets:
2 mg, 3 mg

NIZATIDINE
ni ZA ti deen
TRADE NAME(S):
Axid AR, Axid
THERAPEUTIC CLASS:
Antiulcer agent
GENERAL USES:
Duodenal ulcer, GERD,
heartburn (OTC)
DOSAGE FORMS:
Tablets: 75 mg; Capsules:
150 mg, 300 mg

NORETHINDRONE
nor eth IN drone
TRADE NAME(S):
Micronor, Nor-QD
THERAPEUTIC CLASS:
Contraceptive (progestin
only)
GENERAL USES:
Contraception
DOSAGE FORMS:
Tablets: 0.35 mg

NORETHINDRONE ACETATE
nor eth IN drone
TRADE NAME(S):
Aygestin
THERAPEUTIC CLASS:
Hormone (progestin)
GENERAL USES:
Amenorrhea,
endometriosis
DOSAGE FORMS:
Tablets: 5 mg

NORFLOXACIN (ORAL)
nor FLOKS a sin

TRADE NAME(S):
Noroxin

THERAPEUTIC CLASS:
Anti-infective

GENERAL USES:
Bacterial infections

DOSAGE FORMS:
Tablets: 400 mg

NORGESTREL
nor JES trel

TRADE NAME(S):
Ovrette

THERAPEUTIC CLASS:
Contraceptive (progestin only)

GENERAL USES:
Contraception

DOSAGE FORMS:
Tablets: 0.075 mg

NORTRIPTYLINE
nor TRIP ti leen

TRADE NAME(S):
Aventyl, Pamelor

THERAPEUTIC CLASS:
Antidepressant

GENERAL USES:
Depression

DOSAGE FORMS:
Capsules: 10 mg, 25 mg, 50 mg, 75 mg; Solution: 10 mg/5 mL

NYSTATIN (ORAL)
nye STAT in

TRADE NAME(S):
Nilstat, Mycostatin

THERAPEUTIC CLASS:
Antifungal

GENERAL USES:
Oral fungal infections (candidiasis)

DOSAGE FORMS:
Suspension: 100,000 units/mL; Troches: 200,000 units; Tablets: 500,000 units

OBINUTUZUMAB
OH bi nyoo TOOZ oo mab

TRADE NAME(S):
Gazyva

THERAPEUTIC CLASS:
Antineoplastic

GENERAL USES:
CLL

DOSAGE FORMS:
Injection: 1000 mg

OCRIPLASMIN
ok ri PLAZ min

TRADE NAME(S):
Jetrea

THERAPEUTIC CLASS:
Ocular agent

GENERAL USES:
Symptomatic vitreomacular adhesion

DOSAGE FORMS:
Injection: 0.5 mg

OCTREOTIDE
ok TREE oh tide
TRADE NAME(S):
Sandostatin, Sandostatin
LAR Depot
THERAPEUTIC CLASS:
Hormone
GENERAL USES:
Acromegaly, carcinoid
tumors
DOSAGE FORMS:
Injection: 0.05 mg,
0.1 mg, 0.5 mg, 1 mg,
5 mg, 10 mg, 20 mg,
30 mg

OFATUMUMAB
oh fuh TOO muh mab
TRADE NAME(S):
Arzerra
THERAPEUTIC CLASS:
Antineoplastic
(monoclonal antibody)
GENERAL USES:
CLL
DOSAGE FORMS:
Injection: 100 mg

OFLOXACIN
oh FLOKS a sin
TRADE NAME(S):
Floxin
THERAPEUTIC CLASS:
Anti-infective
GENERAL USES:
Bacterial infections

DOSAGE FORMS:
Tablets: 200 mg, 300 mg,
400 mg; Injection:
200 mg, 400 mg

OFLOXACIN (OCULAR)
oh FLOKS a sin
TRADE NAME(S):
Ocuflox
THERAPEUTIC CLASS:
Ocular agent
(anti-infective)
GENERAL USES:
Ocular infections
DOSAGE FORMS:
Ophthalmic solution:
3 mg/mL

OFLOXACIN (OTIC)
oh FLOKS a sin
TRADE NAME(S):
Floxin Otic
THERAPEUTIC CLASS:
Anti-infective (otic)
GENERAL USES:
Otitis externa
DOSAGE FORMS:
Otic solution: 0.3%

OLANZAPINE
oh LAN za peen
TRADE NAME(S):
Zyprexa, Zyprexa Relprevv
THERAPEUTIC CLASS:
Antipsychotic
GENERAL USES:
Psychotic disorders

DOSAGE FORMS:
Tablets: 2.5 mg,
5 mg, 7.5 mg, 10 mg,
15 mg, 20 mg; Orally
disintegrating tablets:
5 mg, 10 mg, 15 mg,
20 mg; Injection:
10 mg, 210 mg, 300 mg,
405 mg

OLANZAPINE/
FLUOXETINE
oh LAN za peen/floo OKS
e teen
TRADE NAME(S):
Symbyax
THERAPEUTIC CLASS:
Antipsychotic/
antidepressant
GENERAL USES:
Bipolar disorder/
depression
DOSAGE FORMS:
Capsules: 6 mg/25 mg,
6 mg/50 mg, 12 mg/
25 mg, 12 mg/50 mg

OLMESARTAN
ole me SAR tan
TRADE NAME(S):
Benicar
THERAPEUTIC CLASS:
Antihypertensive
GENERAL USES:
Hypertension
DOSAGE FORMS:
Tablets: 5 mg, 20 mg,
40 mg

OLMESARTAN/HCTZ
ole me SAR tan/hye droe
klor oh THYE a zide
TRADE NAME(S):
Benicar HCT
THERAPEUTIC CLASS:
Antihypertensive/
diuretic
GENERAL USES:
Hypertension
DOSAGE FORMS:
Tablets: 20 mg/12.5 mg,
40 mg/12.5 mg, 40 mg/
25 mg

OLODATEROL
OH loe DA ter ol
TRADE NAME(S):
Striverdi Respimat
THERAPEUTIC CLASS:
Bronchodilator
GENERAL USES:
COPD
DOSAGE FORMS:
Inhalation: 2.5 mcg/
inhalation

OLOPATADINE (NASAL)
oh la PAT a deen
TRADE NAME(S):
Patanase
THERAPEUTIC CLASS:
Nasal agent
GENERAL USES:
Seasonal allergies
DOSAGE FORMS:
Nasal spray: 665 mcg/
spray

OLOPATADINE (OCULAR)
oh la PAT a deen

TRADE NAME(S):
Patanol

THERAPEUTIC CLASS:
Ocular agent

GENERAL USES:
Allergic conjunctivitis

DOSAGE FORMS:
Ophthalmic solution: 0.1%

OLSALAZINE
ol SAL a zeen

TRADE NAME(S):
Dipentum

THERAPEUTIC CLASS:
GI agent

GENERAL USES:
Ulcerative colitis

DOSAGE FORMS:
Capsules: 250 mg

OMALIZUMAB
oh mah lye ZOO mab

TRADE NAME(S):
Xolair

THERAPEUTIC CLASS:
Antiasthma

GENERAL USES:
Asthma, chronic idiopathic urticaria

DOSAGE FORMS:
Injection: 150 mg

OMACETAXINE MEPESUCCINATE
OH ma se TAX een

TRADE NAME(S):
Synribo

THERAPEUTIC CLASS:
Antineoplastic

GENERAL USES:
CML

DOSAGE FORMS:
Injection: 3.5 mg

OMEGA-3 ACID ETHYL ESTERS
oh MEG a three AS id ETH il ES ters

TRADE NAME(S):
Lovaza, Omtryg

THERAPEUTIC CLASS:
Fish oil

GENERAL USES:
Hypertriglyceridemia

DOSAGE FORMS:
Capsules: 1 g, 1.2 g

OMEGA-3-CARBOXYLIC ACIDS
Oh MEG a three kar BOKS il ik AS ids

TRADE NAME(S):
Epanova

THERAPEUTIC CLASS:
Fish oil

GENERAL USES:
Hypertriglyceridemia

DOSAGE FORMS:
Capsules: 1 g

OMEPRAZOLE
oh MEP ra zole

TRADE NAME(S):
Prilosec

THERAPEUTIC CLASS:
Gastric acid secretion inhibitor

GENERAL USES:
Duodenal ulcer, GERD

DOSAGE FORMS:
Delayed-release capsules: 10 mg, 20 mg, 40 mg; Oral suspension: 20 mg

OMEPRAZOLE/SODIUM BICARBONATE
oh MEP ra zole/SOE dee um bye KAR bo nate

TRADE NAME(S):
Zegerid

THERAPEUTIC CLASS:
Gastric acid secretion inhibitor/anti-ulcer agent

GENERAL USES:
Duodenal ulcer, gastric ulcer, GERD, erosive esophagitis

DOSAGE FORMS:
Capsules: 20 mg/ 1100 mg, 40 mg/ 1100 mg; Oral suspension (powder): 20 mg/1680 mg, 40 mg/ 1680 mg

ONABOTULINUMTOXINA
OH na BOT yoo li num TOKS in A

TRADE NAME(S):
Botox, Botox Cosmetic

THERAPEUTIC CLASS:
Toxoid

GENERAL USES:
Cervical dystonia, severe underarm sweating, strabismus, eyelid tics; facial wrinkles; chronic migraine headaches; overactive bladder

DOSAGE FORMS:
Injection: 50 units, 100 units, 200 units

ONDANSETRON
on DAN se tron

TRADE NAME(S):
Zofran, Zuplenz

THERAPEUTIC CLASS:
Antiemetic

GENERAL USES:
Surgical or chemotherapy nausea/vomiting

DOSAGE FORMS:
Tablets: 4 mg, 8 mg, 24 mg; Solution: 4 mg/ 5 mL; Orally disintegrating tablets: 4 mg, 8 mg; Injection: 4 mg, 80 mg; Oral soluble film: 4 mg, 8 mg

ORITAVANCIN
OR eh ta VAN sin

TRADE NAME(S):
Orbactiv

THERAPEUTIC CLASS:
  Anti-infective
GENERAL CLASS:
  Bacterial infections
DOSAGE FORMS:
  Injection: 400 mg

ORLISTAT
OR li stat
TRADE NAME(S):
  Xenical
THERAPEUTIC CLASS:
  Anti-obesity
GENERAL USES:
  Obesity
DOSAGE FORMS:
  Capsules: 120 mg

ORPHENADRINE
or FEN a dreen
TRADE NAME(S):
  Norflex
THERAPEUTIC CLASS:
  Skeletal muscle relaxant
GENERAL USES:
  Musculoskeletal
  conditions
DOSAGE FORMS:
  Tablets and Sustained-
  release tablets: 100 mg

OSELTAMIVIR
oh sel TAM i veer
TRADE NAME(S):
  Tamiflu
THERAPEUTIC CLASS:
  Anti-influenza

GENERAL USES:
  Influenza A or B
DOSAGE FORMS:
  Capsules: 30 mg, 45 mg,
  75 mg; Oral suspension:
  12 mg/mL

OSPEMIFENE
os PEM i feen
TRADE NAME(S):
  Osphena
THERAPEUTIC CLASS:
  Estrogen agonist/
  antagonist
GENERAL USES:
  Symptoms of menopause
DOSAGE FORMS:
  Tablets: 60 mg

OXACILLIN
oks a SIL in
TRADE NAME(S):
  Oxacillin
THERAPEUTIC CLASS:
  Anti-infective
GENERAL USES:
  Bacterial infections
DOSAGE FORMS:
  Capsules: 250 mg,
  500 mg; Solution:
  250 mg/5 mL; Injection:
  250 mg, 500 mg, 1 g, 2 g,
  4 g, 10 g

OXALIPLATIN
oks AL i pla tin
TRADE NAME(S):
  Eloxatin

THERAPEUTIC CLASS:
Antineoplastic

GENERAL USES:
Colon or rectal cancer (metastatic)

DOSAGE FORMS:
Injection: 50 mg, 100 mg

OXAPROZIN
oks a PROE zin

TRADE NAME(S):
Daypro

THERAPEUTIC CLASS:
Anti-inflammatory/ analgesic

GENERAL USES:
Osteoarthritis, rheumatoid arthritis

DOSAGE FORMS:
Tablets: 600 mg

OXAZEPAM
oks A ze pam

TRADE NAME(S):
Serax

THERAPEUTIC CLASS:
Antianxiety agent

GENERAL USES:
Anxiety

DOSAGE FORMS:
Tablets: 15 mg; Capsules: 10 mg, 15 mg, 30 mg

OXCARBAZEPINE
oks car BAZ e peen

TRADE NAME(S):
Trileptal, Oxtellar XR

THERAPEUTIC CLASS:
Anticonvulsant

GENERAL USES:
Partial seizures

DOSAGE FORMS:
Tablets: 150 mg, 300 mg, 600 mg; Extended-release tablets: 150 mg, 300 mg, 600 mg; Suspension: 300 mg/5 mL

OXYBATE, SODIUM
OKS i bate

TRADE NAME(S):
Xyrem

THERAPEUTIC CLASS:
CNS depressant

GENERAL USES:
Cataplexy in narcolepsy

DOSAGE FORMS:
Solution: 500 mg/mL

OXYBUTYNIN
oks i BYOO ti nin

TRADE NAME(S):
Ditropan, Ditropan XL

THERAPEUTIC CLASS:
Antispasmodic

GENERAL USES:
Bladder instability

DOSAGE FORMS:
Tablets: 5 mg; Extended-release tablets: 5 mg, 10 mg, 15 mg; Syrup: 5 mg/5 mL

**OXYBUTYNIN
(TRANSDERMAL)**
oks i BYOO ti nin
TRADE NAME(S):
Oxytrol, Gelnique
THERAPEUTIC CLASS:
Antispasmodic
GENERAL USES:
Bladder instability
DOSAGE FORMS:
Gel: 10%; Patch: 3.9 mg

OXYCODONE
oks i KOE done
TRADE NAME(S):
Percolone, Roxicodone,
Oxecta, OxyContin,
OxyIR, OxyFast
THERAPEUTIC CLASS:
Analgesic (narcotic)
GENERAL USES:
Pain
DOSAGE FORMS:
Tablets: 5 mg, 7.5 mg;
Capsules: 5 mg;
Controlled-release tablets:
10 mg, 20 mg, 40 mg,
80 mg; Solution: 5 mg/5 mL;
Concentrated solution:
20 mg/mL

**OXYCODONE/
ACETAMINOPHEN**
oks i KOE done/a seet a MIN
oh fen
TRADE NAME(S):
Endocet, Percocet,
Roxicet, Xartemis XR

THERAPEUTIC CLASS:
Analgesic
GENERAL USES:
Pain
DOSAGE FORMS:
Tablets: 2.5 mg/325 mg,
5 mg/325 mg, 7.5 mg/325
mg, 10 mg/325 mg;
Extended-release tablets:
7.5 mg/325 mg; Solution:
5 mg/325 mg per 5 mL

OXYCODONE/NALOXONE
oks i KOE done/nal AKS one
TRADE NAME(S):
Targiniq ER
THERAPEUTIC CLASS:
Analgesic (narcotic)/
antidote
GENERAL USES:
Pain
DOSAGE FORMS:
Extended-release tablets:
10 mg/5 mg, 20 mg/10
mg, 40 mg/20 mg

OXYMORPHONE
oks ee MOR fone
TRADE NAME(S):
Opana, Opana ER
THERAPEUTIC CLASS:
Narcotic analgesic
GENERAL USES:
Pain
DOSAGE FORMS:
Tablets: 5 mg, 10 mg;
Extended-release tablets:

5 mg, 7.5 mg, 10 mg,
15 mg, 20 mg, 30 mg,
40 mg; Injection: 1 mg

OXYTOCIN
oks i TOE sin
TRADE NAME(S):
Pitocin, Syntocinon
THERAPEUTIC CLASS:
Oxytocic
GENERAL USES:
Stimulant for labor
DOSAGE FORMS:
Injection: 5 units,
10 units,
100 units

PACLITAXEL
PAK li taks el
TRADE NAME(S):
Taxol
THERAPEUTIC CLASS:
Antineoplastic
GENERAL USES:
Various cancers
DOSAGE FORMS:
Injection: 30 mg,
100.2 mg, 150 mg,
300 mg

**PACLITAXEL
(PROTEIN BOUND)**
PAK li taks el
TRADE NAME(S):
Abraxane
THERAPEUTIC CLASS:
Antineoplastic

GENERAL USES:
Breast cancer, lung
cancer, pancreatic cancer
DOSAGE FORMS:
Injection: 100 mg

PALIFERMIN
pal ee FER min
TRADE NAME(S):
Kepivance
THERAPEUTIC CLASS:
Keratinocyte growth factor
GENERAL USES:
Mucositis
DOSAGE FORMS:
Injection: 6.25 mg

PALIPERIDONE
pal ee PER i done
TRADE NAME(S):
Invega, Invega Sustenna
THERAPEUTIC CLASS:
Atypical antipsychotic
GENERAL USES:
Schizophrenia
DOSAGE FORMS:
Extended-release tablets:
3 mg, 6 mg, 9 mg;
Injection: 39 mg, 78 mg,
117 mg, 156 mg, 234 mg

PALIVIZUMAB
pah li VIZ yoo mab
TRADE NAME(S):
Synagis
THERAPEUTIC CLASS:
Antiviral antibody
GENERAL USES:
RSV prevention

Dosage Forms:
Injection: 50 mg, 100 mg

PALONOSETRON
pal oh NOE se tron
Trade Name(s):
Aloxi
Therapeutic Class:
Antiemetic
General Uses:
Chemotherapy-induced
nausea/vomiting
Dosage Forms:
Capsules: 0.5 mg;
Injection: 0.25 mg

PANCRELIPASE
**(AMYLASE/LIPASE/
PROTEASE)**
pan cre LYE pase
Trade Name(s):
Creon
Therapeutic Class:
Pancreatic enzymes
General Uses:
Pancreatic insufficiency
Dosage Forms:
Delayed-release capsules:
15,000/3,000/9,500
USP units,
30,000/6,000/19,000
USP units,
60,000/12,000/38,000
USP units,
120,000/24,000/76,000
USP units

PANCRELIPASE
**(AMYLASE/LIPASE/
PROTEASE)**
pan cre LYE pase
Trade Name(s):
Pertzye
Therapeutic Class:
Pancreatic enzymes
General Uses:
Pancreatic insufficiency
Dosage Forms:
Delayed-release capsules:
30,250/8,000/28,750
USP units,
60,500/16,000/57,500
USP units

PANCRELIPASE
**(AMYLASE/LIPASE/
PROTEASE)**
pan cre LYE pase
Trade Name(s):
Ultresa
Therapeutic Class:
Pancreatic enzymes
General Uses:
Pancreatic insufficiency
Dosage Forms:
Delayed-release capsules:
27,600/13,800/27,600
USP units,
41,400/20,700/41,400
USP units,
46,000/23,000/46,000
USP units

PANCRELIPASE
(AMYLASE/LIPASE/
PROTEASE)
pan cre LYE pase

TRADE NAME(S):
Viokace

THERAPEUTIC CLASS:
Pancreatic enzymes

GENERAL USES:
Pancreatic insufficiency

DOSAGE FORMS:
Tablets:
39,150/10,440/39,150
USP units,
78,300/20,880/78,300
USP units

PANCURONIUM
pan kyoo ROE nee um

TRADE NAME(S):
Pavulon

THERAPEUTIC CLASS:
Muscle relaxant

GENERAL USES:
Muscle relaxation for
intubation

DOSAGE FORMS:
Injection: 4 mg, 10 mg

PANITUMUMAB
pan ee TOO myoo mab

TRADE NAME(S):
Vectibix

THERAPEUTIC CLASS:
Antineoplastic

GENERAL USES:
Colon cancer

DOSAGE FORMS:
Injection: 100 mg,
200 mg, 400 mg

PANTOPRAZOLE
pan TOE pra zole

TRADE NAME(S):
Protonix

THERAPEUTIC CLASS:
Gastric acid secretion
inhibitor

GENERAL USES:
Erosive esophagitis, GERD

DOSAGE FORMS:
Delayed-release tablets:
20 mg, 40 mg; Injection:
40 mg; Delayed-release
granules: 40 mg

PAPAVERINE
pa PAV er een

TRADE NAME(S):
Pavabid, Pavacot

THERAPEUTIC CLASS:
Cardiac agent

GENERAL USES:
Peripheral and cerebral
ischemia

DOSAGE FORMS:
Sustained-release
capsules: 150 mg

PARICALCITOL
pah ri KAL si tole

TRADE NAME(S):
Zemplar

THERAPEUTIC CLASS:
    Vitamin D analog
GENERAL USES:
    Secondary
    hyperparathyroidism in
    kidney disease
    (children)
DOSAGE FORMS:
    Injection: 2 mcg, 5 mcg,
    10 mcg; Capsules: 1 mcg,
    2 mcg, 4 mcg

PAROMOMYCIN
par oh moe MYE sin
TRADE NAME(S):
    Humatin
THERAPEUTIC CLASS:
    Antituberculosis
    agent
GENERAL USES:
    Tuberculosis
DOSAGE FORMS:
    Capsules: 250 mg

PAROXETINE
pa ROKS e teen
TRADE NAME(S):
    Paxil, Paxil CR,
    Asimia, Brisdelle
THERAPEUTIC CLASS:
    Antidepressant
GENERAL USES:
    Depression, OCD, panic,
    social anxiety, PMDD,
    PTSD, menopause
DOSAGE FORMS:
    Tablets: 10 mg,

20 mg, 30 mg, 40 mg;
Controlled-release tablets:
12.5 mg, 25 mg, 37.5 mg;
Capsules: 7.5 mg;
Suspension: 10 mg/5 mL

**PASIREOTIDE
DIASPARTATE**
PAS i REE oh tide
TRADE NAME(S):
    Signifor
THERAPEUTIC CLASS:
    Somatostatin
GENERAL USES:
    Cushing's disease
DOSAGE FORMS:
    Injection: 0.3 mg, 0.6 mg,
    0.9 mg

PAZOPANIB
paz OH pa nib
TRADE NAME(S):
    Votrient
THERAPEUTIC CLASS:
    Antineoplastic
GENERAL USES:
    Renal cell carcinoma, soft
    tissue sarcoma
DOSAGE FORMS:
    Tablets: 200 mg

PEGAPTANIB SODIUM
peg AP ta nib
TRADE NAME(S):
    Macugen
THERAPEUTIC CLASS:
    Ocular agent

GENERAL USES:
Macular degeneration
DOSAGE FORMS:
Injection: 0.3 mg

PEGFILGRASTIM
PEG fil GRAS tim
TRADE NAME(S):
Neulasta
THERAPEUTIC CLASS:
Blood cell stimulator
GENERAL USES:
Prevent infection in
cancer patients
DOSAGE FORMS:
Injection: 6 mg

PEGINESATIDE ACETATE
PEG in ES a tide AS e tate
TRADE NAME(S):
Omontys, Omontys PF
THERAPEUTIC CLASS:
Hematological agent
GENERAL USES:
Anemia with chronic renal
failure
DOSAGE FORMS:
Injection: 10 mg, 20 mg;
PF injection: 1 mg, 2 mg,
3 mg, 4 mg, 5 mg, 6 mg

PEGINTERFERON ALFA-2a
peg in ter FEER on
TRADE NAME(S):
Pegasys
THERAPEUTIC CLASS:
Antiviral

GENERAL USES:
Hepatitis C
DOSAGE FORMS:
Injection: 180 mcg

PEGINTERFERON ALFA-2b
peg in ter FEER on
TRADE NAME(S):
Peg-Intron, Sylatron
THERAPEUTIC CLASS:
Antiviral, antineoplastic
GENERAL USES:
Hepatitis C, melanoma
DOSAGE FORMS:
Injection: 50 mcg,
80 mcg, 120 mcg,
150 mcg, 296 mcg,
444 mcg, 888 mcg

PEGINTERFERON BETA-1A
peg in ter FEER on BAY ta
TRADE NAME(S):
Plegridy
THERAPEUTIC CLASS:
Immunological agent
GENERAL CLASS:
MS
DOSAGE FORMS:
Injection: 63 mcg, 94
mcg, 125 mcg

PEGLOTICASE
peg LOE ti kase
TRADE NAME(S):
Krystexxa

THERAPEUTIC CLASS:
Uric acid inihibitor

GENERAL USES:
Chronic gout

DOSAGE FORMS:
Injection: 8 mg

PEGVISOMANT
peg VYE soe mant

TRADE NAME(S):
Somavert

THERAPEUTIC CLASS:
Growth hormone antagonist

GENERAL USES:
Acromegaly

DOSAGE FORMS:
Injection: 10 mg, 15 mg, 20 mg

PEMBROLIZUMAB
pem broe lye ZOO mab

TRADE NAME(S):
Keytruda

THERAPEUTIC CLASS:
Antineoplastic

GENERAL CLASS:
Metastatic melanoma

DOSAGE FORMS:
Injection: 50 mg

PEMETREXED
pem e TREKS ed

TRADE NAME(S):
Alimta

THERAPEUTIC CLASS:
Antineoplastic

GENERAL USES:
Various lung cancers

DOSAGE FORMS:
Injection: 500 mg

PENBUTOLOL
pen BYOO toe lole

TRADE NAME(S):
Levatol

THERAPEUTIC CLASS:
Antihypertensive

GENERAL USES:
Hypertension

DOSAGE FORMS:
Tablets: 20 mg

PENCICLOVIR
pen SYE kloe veer

TRADE NAME(S):
Denavir

THERAPEUTIC CLASS:
Antiviral (topical)

GENERAL USES:
Cold sores, oral herpes

DOSAGE FORMS:
Cream: 1%

PENICILLIN G (AQUEOUS)
pen i SIL in

TRADE NAME(S):
Penicillin G Potassium, Pfizerpen

THERAPEUTIC CLASS:
Anti-infective

GENERAL USES:
Bacterial infections

DOSAGE FORMS:
Injection: 1 million units,
2 million units, 3 million
units, 5 million units,
10 million units, 20 million
units

PENICILLIN G BENZATHINE
pen i SIL in jee BENZ a theen
TRADE NAME(S):
Bicillin LA, Permapen
THERAPEUTIC CLASS:
Anti-infective
GENERAL USES:
Bacterial infections
DOSAGE FORMS:
Injection: 600,000 units,
1.2 million units,
2.4 million units,
3 million units

PENICILLIN G PROCAINE
pen i SIL in jee PROE kane
TRADE NAME(S):
Wycillin
THERAPEUTIC CLASS:
Anti-infective
GENERAL USES:
Bacterial infections
DOSAGE FORMS:
Injection: 600,000 units,
1.2 million units,
2.4 million units

PENICILLIN VK
pen i SIL in
TRADE NAME(S):
Beepen-VK,
Pen-Vee K, Veetids
THERAPEUTIC CLASS:
Anti-infective
GENERAL USES:
Bacterial infections
DOSAGE FORMS:
Tablets: 250 mg, 500 mg;
Solution: 125 mg/5 mL,
250 mg/5 mL

PENTAMIDINE ISETHIONATE
pen TAM i deen ice e THYE ah nate
TRADE NAME(S):
Pentam 300, NebuPent
THERAPEUTIC CLASS:
Anti-infective
GENERAL USES:
Treatment or prevention
of pneumonia in HIV
infection
DOSAGE FORMS:
Injection and Aerosol:
300 mg

PENTETATE CALCIUM TRISODIUM
PEN te tate
TRADE NAME(S):
Ca-DTPA
THERAPEUTIC CLASS:
Antidote

GENERAL USES:
Internal contamination with plutonium, americium, curium

DOSAGE FORMS:
Injection or Inhalation: 1000 mg

PENTETATE ZINC TRISODIUM
PEN te tate

TRADE NAME(S):
Zn-DTPA

THERAPEUTIC CLASS:
Antidote

GENERAL USES:
Internal contamination with plutonium, americium, curium

DOSAGE FORMS:
Injection: 1000 mg

PENTOBARBITAL
pen toe BAR bi tal

TRADE NAME(S):
Nembutal

THERAPEUTIC CLASS:
Sedative/hypnotic

GENERAL USES:
Insomnia (short-term therapy), pre-op sedative

DOSAGE FORMS:
Capsules: 50 mg, 100 mg; Elixir: 18.2 mg/5 mL; Injection: 1 g, 2.5 g

PENTOXIFYLLINE
pen toks I fi leen

TRADE NAME(S):
Pentoxil, Trental

THERAPEUTIC CLASS:
Blood viscosity reducer agent

GENERAL USES:
Intermittent claudication

DOSAGE FORMS:
Tablets, Controlled-release tablets, Extended-release tablets: 400 mg

PERAMPANEL
per AM pa nel

TRADE NAME(S):
Fycompa

THERAPEUTIC CLASS:
Anticonvulsant

GENERAL USES:
Partial seizures

DOSAGE FORMS:
Tablets: 2 mg, 4 mg, 6 mg, 8 mg, 10 mg, 12 mg

PERMETHRIN
per METH rin

TRADE NAME(S):
Elimite, Acticin, Nix

THERAPEUTIC CLASS:
Scabicide/pediculicide (topical)

GENERAL USES:
Scabies, head lice

DOSAGE FORMS:
Cream: 5%; Lotion: 1%

PERPHENAZINE
per FEN a zeen
TRADE NAME(S):
Trilafon
THERAPEUTIC CLASS:
Antipsychotic
GENERAL USES:
Psychotic disorders
DOSAGE FORMS:
Tablets: 2 mg, 4 mg,
8 mg, 16 mg;
Concentrated
solution: 16 mg/5 mL;
Injection: 5 mg

**PERPHENAZINE/
AMITRIPTYLINE**
per FEN a zeen/a mee TRIP
ti leen
TRADE NAME(S):
Etrafon, Triavil
THERAPEUTIC CLASS:
Sedative/antidepressant
GENERAL USES:
Depression/anxiety
DOSAGE FORMS:
Tablets: 2 mg/10 mg,
2 mg/25 mg, 4 mg/
25 mg, 4 mg/50 mg

PERTUZUMAB
per TOOZ oo mab
TRADE NAME(S):
Perjeta
THERAPEUTIC CLASS:
Antineoplastic
GENERAL USES:
Breast cancer

DOSAGE FORMS:
Injection: 420 mg

PHENELZINE
FEN el zeen
TRADE NAME(S):
Nardil
THERAPEUTIC CLASS:
Antidepressant
GENERAL USES:
Depression
DOSAGE FORMS:
Tablets: 15 mg

PHENOBARBITAL
fee noe BAR bi tal
TRADE NAME(S):
Barbita, Solfoton
THERAPEUTIC CLASS:
Sedative/hypnotic,
anticonvulsant
GENERAL USES:
Seizures, insomnia
(short-term
therapy)
DOSAGE FORMS:
Tablets: 8 mg, 15 mg,
16 mg, 30 mg, 60 mg,
90 mg, 100 mg; Capsules:
16 mg; Elixir: 15 mg/
5 mL, 20 mg/5 mL;
Injection: 60 mg, 65 mg,
130 mg

PHENTERMINE
FEN ter meen
TRADE NAME(S):
Fastin, Zantryl, Adipex-P,

Ionamin, Suprenza

THERAPEUTIC CLASS:
Anorexiant

GENERAL USES:
Obesity

DOSAGE FORMS:
Tablets: 8 mg, 37.5 mg;
Capsules: 15 mg,
18.75 mg, 30 mg, 37.5 mg;
Orally disintegrating
tablets: 15 mg, 30 mg,
37.5 mg

PHENTERMINE/
TOPIRAMATE
FEN ter meen/toe PYRE a
mate

TRADE NAME(S):
Qsymia

THERAPEUTIC CLASS:
Anorexiant

GENERAL USES:
Obesity

DOSAGE FORMS:
Extended-release
capsules: 3.75 mg/23 mg,
7.5 mg/46 mg, 11.25 mg/
69 mg, 15 mg/92 mg

PHENYLEPHRINE HCL
fen ill EFF rin

TRADE NAME(S):
Vazculep

THERAPEUTIC CLASS:
Sympathomimetic

GENERAL USES:
Hypotension, shock

DOSAGE FORMS:
Injection: 10 mg, 50 mg,
100 mg

PHENYLEPHRINE HCL
(OCULAR)
fen ill EFF rin

TRADE NAME(S):
Phenylephrine HCL

THERAPEUTIC CLASS:
Ocular agent

GENERAL USES:
Pupil dilation

DOSAGE FORMS:
Ophthalmic solution:
2.5%, 10%

PHENYTOIN
FEN i toyn

TRADE NAME(S):
Dilantin

THERAPEUTIC CLASS:
Anticonvulsant

GENERAL USES:
Seizures

DOSAGE FORMS:
Chewable tablets: 50 mg;
Suspension: 125 mg/
5 mL; Extended-release
tablets: 30 mg, 100 mg;
Prompt capsules: 100 mg;
Injection: 100 mg, 250 mg

PILOCARPINE (OCULAR)
pye loe KAR peen

TRADE NAME(S):
Isopto Carpine, Pilocar,

Akarpine, Pilostat

THERAPEUTIC CLASS:
Ocular agent

GENERAL USES:
Glaucoma

DOSAGE FORMS:
Ophthalmic solution:
0.25%, 0.5%, 1%, 2%,
3%, 4%, 5%, 6%, 8%,
10%;

PILOCARPINE (ORAL)
pye loe KAR peen

TRADE NAME(S):
Salagen

THERAPEUTIC CLASS:
Saliva stimulant

GENERAL USES:
Saliva deficiency

DOSAGE FORMS:
Tablets: 5 mg

PIMECROLIMUS
pim e KROE li mus

TRADE NAME(S):
Elidel

THERAPEUTIC CLASS:
Anti-inflammatory agent

GENERAL USES:
Eczema

DOSAGE FORMS:
Cream: 1%

PIMOZIDE
PI moe zide

TRADE NAME(S):
Orap

THERAPEUTIC CLASS:
Antipsychotic

GENERAL USES:
Tourette's

DOSAGE FORMS:
Tablets: 2 mg

PINDOLOL
PIN doe lole

TRADE NAME(S):
Visken

THERAPEUTIC CLASS:
Antihypertensive

GENERAL USES:
Hypertension

DOSAGE FORMS:
Tablets: 5 mg, 10 mg

PIOGLITAZONE
pye oh GLI ta zone

TRADE NAME(S):
Actos

THERAPEUTIC CLASS:
Antidiabetic

GENERAL USES:
Diabetes (type 2)

DOSAGE FORMS:
Tablets: 15 mg, 30 mg,
45 mg

PIOGLITAZONE/ GLIMEPIRIDE
pye oh GLI ta zone/glye MEP i ride

TRADE NAME(S):
Duetact

THERAPEUTIC CLASS:
Antidiabetic

GENERAL USES:
Diabetes (type 2)
DOSAGE FORMS:
Tablets: 30 mg/2 mg,
30 mg/4 mg

PIPERACILLIN
pi PER a sil in
TRADE NAME(S):
Pipracil
THERAPEUTIC CLASS:
Anti-infective
GENERAL USES:
Bacterial infections
DOSAGE FORMS:
Injection: 2 g, 3 g, 4 g,
40 g

PIPERACILLIN/ TAZOBACTAM
pi PER a sil in/ta zoe BAK tam
TRADE NAME(S):
Zosyn
THERAPEUTIC CLASS:
Anti-infective
GENERAL USES:
Bacterial infections
DOSAGE FORMS:
Injection: 2 g/0.25 g,
3 g/0.375 g, 4 g/0.5 g,
36 g/4.5 g

PIRBUTEROL
peer BYOO ter ole
TRADE NAME(S):
Maxair
THERAPEUTIC CLASS:
Bronchodilator
GENERAL USES:
Bronchospasm, asthma
DOSAGE FORMS:
Inhaler: 0.2 mg/inhalation

PIROXICAM
peer OKS i kam
TRADE NAME(S):
Feldene
THERAPEUTIC CLASS:
Anti-inflammatory/
analgesic
GENERAL USES:
Osteoarthritis, rheumatoid
arthritis
DOSAGE FORMS:
Capsules: 10 mg, 20 mg

PITAVASTATIN CALCIUM
pih TAH va stat in
TRADE NAME(S):
Livalo
THERAPEUTIC CLASS:
Antilipemic
GENERAL USES:
Hyperlipidemia
DOSAGE FORMS:
Tablets: 1 mg, 2 mg, 4 mg

PLERIXAFOR
pler IX a fore
TRADE NAME(S):
Mozobil
THERAPEUTIC CLASS:
Hematological agent
GENERAL USES:
Non-Hodgkin's
lymphoma, multiple
myeloma

DOSAGE FORMS:
Injection: 24 mg

POLIDOCANOL
pol ee DOE ka nole
TRADE NAME(S):
Asclera, Varithena
THERAPEUTIC CLASS:
Sclerosing agent
GENERAL USES:
Varicose veins
DOSAGE FORMS:
Injection: 0.5%, 1%

POLYETHYLENE GLYCOL
pol ee ETH i leen GLY kol
TRADE NAME(S):
MiraLax, GlycoLax
THERAPEUTIC CLASS:
Laxative
GENERAL USES:
Bowel cleansing
DOSAGE FORMS:
Powder for oral solution:
255 g, 527 g

**POLYETHYLENE GLYCOL
3350/SODIUM SULFATE/
POTASSIUM SULFATE/
MAGNESIUM SULFATE/
SODIUM CHLORIDE/
SODIUM BICARBONATE/
POTASSIUM CHLORIDE**
pall ee ETH il een GLYE kol/
SOE dee um SUL fate /poe
TASS ee um SUL fate/mag
NEE zhum SUL fate /SOE

dee um KLOR id/SOE de um
bye KARB i nate/poe TASS
ee um KLOR id
TRADE NAME(S):
Suclear
THERAPEUTIC CLASS:
Bowel preparation
GENERAL USES:
Preparation for
colonoscopy
DOSAGE FORMS:
Solution: 210 g PEG-
3350/5.6 g sodium
chloride/2.86 g sodium
bicarbonate/0.74 g
potassium chloride

POLY-UREA URETHANE
pol ee YOO re a YUR a thane
TRADE NAME(S):
Nuvail
THERAPEUTIC CLASS:
Nail protectant
GENERAL USES:
Nail dystrophy, damaged
nails
DOSAGE FORMS:
Solution: 16%

POMALIDOMIDE
pom a LID oh mide
TRADE NAME(S):
Pomalyst
THERAPEUTIC CLASS:
Antineoplastic
GENERAL USES:
Multiple myeloma

DOSAGE FORMS:
Capsules: 1 mg, 2 mg, 3 mg, 4 mg

PONATINIB
poe NA ti nib
TRADE NAME(S):
Iclusig
THERAPEUTIC CLASS:
Antineoplastic
GENERAL USES:
ALL, CML
DOSAGE FORMS:
Tablets: 15 mg, 45 mg

POSACONAZOLE
poe sa KON a zole
TRADE NAME(S):
Noxafil
THERAPEUTIC CLASS:
Antifungal
GENERAL USES:
Fungal infections
DOSAGE FORMS:
Delayed-release tablets: 100 mg; Injection: 300 mg; Oral suspension: 40 mg/mL

POTASSIUM CHLORIDE
poe TASS ee um KLOR ide
TRADE NAME(S):
K-Dur, Kaon-Cl, Klor-Con, Klotrix, Klorvess, K-Lyte, Micro-K
THERAPEUTIC CLASS:
Electrolyte (potassium)

GENERAL USES:
Potassium replacement
DOSAGE FORMS:
Controlled-release or Extended-release tablets: 6.7 mEq, 8 mEq, 10 mEq; Effervescent tablets: 20 mEq, 25 mEq, 50 mEq; Liquid: 20 mEq, 30 mEq or 40 mEq/15 mL; Powder: 20 mEq, 25 mEq; Injection: various concentrations

PRALATREXATE
PRAL a TREX ate
TRADE NAME(S):
Folotyn
THERAPEUTIC CLASS:
Antineoplastic
GENERAL USES:
T-cell lymphoma
DOSAGE FORMS:
Injection: 20 mg, 40 mg

PRAMIPEXOLE
pra mi PEKS ole
TRADE NAME(S):
Mirapex, Mirapex ER
THERAPEUTIC CLASS:
Antiparkinson agent
GENERAL USES:
Parkinson's disease
DOSAGE FORMS:
Tablets: 0.125 mg, 0.25 mg, 0.5 mg, 0.75 mg, 1 mg, 1.5 mg; Extended-

release tablets: 0.375 mg, 0.75 mg, 1.5 mg, 3 mg, 4.5 mg

PRAMLINTIDE ACETATE
PRAM lin tide

TRADE NAME(S):
Symlin

THERAPEUTIC CLASS:
Antidiabetic

GENERAL USES:
Diabetes

DOSAGE FORMS:
Injection: 3 mg

PRASUGREL
PRA soo grel

TRADE NAME(S):
Effient

THERAPEUTIC CLASS:
Antiplatelet agent

GENERAL USES:
Reduce thrombotic risk in acute coronary syndrome

DOSAGE FORMS:
Tablets: 5 mg, 10 mg

PRAVASTATIN
PRA va stat in

TRADE NAME(S):
Pravachol

THERAPEUTIC CLASS:
Antilipemic

GENERAL USES:
Hyperlipidemia

DOSAGE FORMS:
Tablets: 10 mg, 20 mg, 40 mg, 80 mg

PRAZOSIN
PRA zoe sin

TRADE NAME(S):
Minipress

THERAPEUTIC CLASS:
Antihypertensive

GENERAL USES:
Hypertension

DOSAGE FORMS:
Capsules: 1 mg, 2 mg, 5 mg

PRAZOSIN/ POLYTHIAZIDE
PRA zoe sin/pol i THYE a zide

TRADE NAME(S):
Minizide

THERAPEUTIC CLASS:
Antihypertensive/diuretic

GENERAL USES:
Hypertension

DOSAGE FORMS:
Capsules: 1 mg/0.5 mg, 2 mg/0.5 mg, 5 mg/ 0.5 mg

PREDNISOLONE (OCULAR)
pred NIS oh lone

TRADE NAME(S):
Pred Mild, Econopred, Pred Forte

THERAPEUTIC CLASS:
Ocular agent (steroid)

GENERAL USES:
Ocular inflammation

DOSAGE FORMS:
Ophthalmic suspension
and Solution: 0.1%,
0.125%

PREDNISOLONE (ORAL)
pred NIS oh lone
TRADE NAME(S):
Orapred ODT, Prelone,
Delta-Cortef, Flo-Pred
THERAPEUTIC CLASS:
Glucocorticoid
GENERAL USES:
Endocrine, skin, blood
disorders; asthma
DOSAGE FORMS:
Orally disintegrating
tablets and Tablets:
5 mg; Syrup and Oral
suspension: 5 mg/5 mL,
15 mg/5 mL

PREDNISONE
PRED ni sone
TRADE NAME(S):
Deltasone, Prednicen-M,
Meticorten, Panasol-S,
Rayos
THERAPEUTIC CLASS:
Glucocorticoid
GENERAL USES:
Allergic reactions,
inflammatory disorders,
neoplasm, endocrine,
skin, and blood disorders
DOSAGE FORMS:
Tablets: 1 mg, 2.5 mg,
5 mg, 10 mg, 20 mg,
50 mg; Delayed-release
tablets: 1 mg, 2 mg, 5 mg;
Syrup and Solution: 5 mg/
5 mL; Concentrated
solution: 5 mg/mL

PREGABALIN
pre GAB a lin
TRADE NAME(S):
Lyrica
THERAPEUTIC CLASS:
Anticonvulsant, analgesic
GENERAL USES:
Neuropathic pain,
fibromyalgia, seizures
DOSAGE FORMS:
Capsules: 25 mg,
50 mg, 75 mg,
100 mg, 150 mg,
200 mg, 225 mg,
300 mg; Oral solution:
20 mg/mL

PRIMAQUINE
PRIM a kween
TRADE NAME(S):
Primaquine
THERAPEUTIC CLASS:
Antimalarial
GENERAL USES:
Malaria treatment
DOSAGE FORMS:
Tablets: 26.3 mg

PRIMIDONE
PRI mi done
TRADE NAME(S):
Mysoline

Therapeutic Class:
Anticonvulsant
General Uses:
Seizures
Dosage Forms:
Tablets: 50 mg, 250 mg;
Suspension: 250 mg/
5 mL

PROBENECID
proe BEN e sid
Trade Name(s):
Benemid, Probalan
Therapeutic Class:
Gout agent
General Uses:
Gout
Dosage Forms:
Tablets: 500 mg

PROCAINAMIDE
proe KANE a mide
Trade Name(s):
Pronestyl,
Procanbid
Therapeutic Class:
Antiarrhythmic
General Uses:
Arrhythmias
Dosage Forms:
Tablets: 250 mg, 375 mg,
500 mg; Sustained-
release tablets: 250 mg,
500 mg, 750 mg,
1000 mg; Capsules:
250 mg, 375 mg, 500 mg;
Injection: 1 g

PROCHLORPERAZINE
proe klor PER a zeen
Trade Name(s):
Compazine
Therapeutic Class:
Antiemetic, antipsychotic
General Uses:
Emesis, psychotic
disorders, anxiety
Dosage Forms:
Tablets: 5 mg, 10 mg,
25 mg; Sustained-release
capsules: 10 mg, 15 mg,
30 mg; Syrup: 5 mg/
5 mL; Injection: 10 mg,
50 mg

PROCYCLIDINE
proe SYE kli deen
Trade Name(s):
Kemadrin
Therapeutic Class:
Antiparkinson agent
General Uses:
Parkinson's disease,
drug-induced
extrapyramidal
disorders
Dosage Forms:
Tablets: 5 mg

PROGESTERONE
proe JES ter one
Trade Name(s):
Prometrium
Therapeutic Class:
Hormone (progesterone)

GENERAL USES:
Amenorrhea, uterine bleeding
DOSAGE FORMS:
Capsules: 100 mg; Vaginal gel: 4%, 8%

PROMETHAZINE
proe METH a zeen
TRADE NAME(S):
Phenergan, Promethegan
THERAPEUTIC CLASS:
Antiemetic, antihistamine
GENERAL USES:
Nausea, sedation, allergies
DOSAGE FORMS:
Tablets and Suppositories: 12.5 mg, 25 mg, 50 mg; Syrup: 6.25 mg/5 mL; Injection: 25 mg, 50 mg

PROPAFENONE
proe pa FEEN one
TRADE NAME(S):
Rythmol
THERAPEUTIC CLASS:
Antiarrhythmic
GENERAL USES:
Arrhythmias, tachycardia
DOSAGE FORMS:
Tablets: 150 mg, 225 mg, 300 mg

PROPANTHELINE
proe PAN the leen
TRADE NAME(S):
Pro-Banthine

THERAPEUTIC CLASS:
GI agent
GENERAL USES:
Peptic ulcer
DOSAGE FORMS:
Tablets: 7.5 mg, 15 mg

PROPRANOLOL
proe PRAN oh lole
TRADE NAME(S):
Inderal, Inderal LA, Betachron ER, Innopran XL, Hemangeol
THERAPEUTIC CLASS:
Cardiac agent, antimigraine
GENERAL USES:
Hypertension, angina, MI, migraines, essential tremor, hemangioma
DOSAGE FORMS:
Tablets: 10 mg, 20 mg, 40 mg, 60 mg, 80 mg, 90 mg; Sustained-release and Extended-release capsules: 60 mg, 80 mg, 120 mg, 160 mg; Solution: 4 mg/mL, 4.28 mg/mL, 8 mg/mL; Concentrated solution: 80 mg/mL; Injection: 1 mg

PROPRANOLOL/HCTZ
proe PRAN oh lole/hye droe klor oh THYE a zide
TRADE NAME(S):
Inderide, Inderide LA

THERAPEUTIC CLASS:
Antihypertensive/diuretic
GENERAL USES:
Hypertension
DOSAGE FORMS:
Tablets: 40 mg/25 mg,
80 mg/25 mg; Long-
acting capsules: 80 mg/
50 mg, 120 mg/50 mg,
160 mg/50 mg

PROPYLTHIOURACIL
proe pil thye oh YOOR a sil
TRADE NAME(S):
Propylthiouracil
THERAPEUTIC CLASS:
Antithyroid agent
GENERAL USES:
Hyperthyroidism
DOSAGE FORMS:
Tablets: 50 mg

PROTRIPTYLINE
proe TRIP ti leen
TRADE NAME(S):
Vivactil
THERAPEUTIC CLASS:
Antidepressant
GENERAL USES:
Depression
DOSAGE FORMS:
Tablets: 5 mg, 10 mg

PYRAZINAMIDE
peer a ZIN a mide
TRADE NAME(S):
Pyrazinamide

THERAPEUTIC CLASS:
Antituberculosis
agent
GENERAL USES:
Tuberculosis
DOSAGE FORMS:
Tablets: 500 mg

QUAZEPAM
KWAY ze pam
TRADE NAME(S):
Doral
THERAPEUTIC CLASS:
Sedative/hypnotic
GENERAL USES:
Insomnia
DOSAGE FORMS:
Tablets: 7.5 mg,
15 mg

QUETIAPINE
kwe TYE a peen
TRADE NAME(S):
Seroquel, Seroquel XR
THERAPEUTIC CLASS:
Antipsychotic
GENERAL USES:
Psychotic disorders
DOSAGE FORMS:
Tablets: 25 mg, 100 mg,
200 mg, 300 mg;
Extended-release tablets:
200 mg, 300 mg, 400 mg

QUINAPRIL
KWIN a pril
TRADE NAME(S):
Accupril

THERAPEUTIC CLASS:
Antihypertensive, cardiac agent

GENERAL USES:
Hypertension, heart failure

DOSAGE FORMS:
Tablets: 5 mg, 10 mg, 20 mg, 40 mg

QUINAPRIL/HCTZ
KWIN a pril/hye droe klor oh THYE a zide

TRADE NAME(S):
Quinaretic, Accuretic

THERAPEUTIC CLASS:
Antihypertensive/ diuretic

GENERAL USES:
Hypertension

DOSAGE FORMS:
Tablets: 10 mg/12.5 mg, 20 mg/12.5 mg, 20 mg/ 25 mg

QUINIDINE GLUCONATE
KWIN i deen

TRADE NAME(S):
Quinaglute, Quinalan

THERAPEUTIC CLASS:
Antiarrhythmic

GENERAL USES:
Atrial fibrillation, tachycardia

DOSAGE FORMS:
Sustained-release tablets: 324 mg; Injection: 800 mg

QUINIDINE SULFATE
KWIN i deen

TRADE NAME(S):
Quinora, Quinidex Extentabs

THERAPEUTIC CLASS:
Antiarrhythmic

GENERAL USES:
Atrial fibrillation, tachycardia

DOSAGE FORMS:
Tablets: 200 mg, 300 mg; Extended-release tablets: 300 mg

QUININE SULFATE
KWYE nine

TRADE NAME(S):
Quinine

THERAPEUTIC CLASS:
Antimalarial

GENERAL USES:
Chloroquine-resistant malaria

DOSAGE FORMS:
Capsules: 200 mg, 260 mg, 325 mg; Tablets: 260 mg

RABEPRAZOLE
ra BEP ra zole

TRADE NAME(S):
Aciphex, Aciphex Sprinkle

THERAPEUTIC CLASS:
Gastric acid secretion inhibitor

GENERAL USES:
GERD, duodenal ulcer,

hyperacidity disorders

DOSAGE FORMS:
Delayed-release tablets:
20 mg; Delayed-release
capsules: 5 mg, 10 mg

RALOXIFENE
ral OKS i feen
TRADE NAME(S):
Evista
THERAPEUTIC CLASS:
Hormone
(estrogen modulator)
GENERAL USES:
Osteoporosis prevention,
breast cancer
DOSAGE FORMS:
Tablets: 60 mg

**RALTEGRAVIR
POTASSIUM**
ral TEG ra veer
TRADE NAME(S):
Isentress
THERAPEUTIC CLASS:
Antiviral
GENERAL USES:
HIV infection
DOSAGE FORMS:
Tablets: 400 mg;
Chewable tablets: 25 mg,
100 mg; Suspension:
100 mg

RAMELTEON
ra MEL tee on
TRADE NAME(S):
Rozerem

THERAPEUTIC CLASS:
Sedative/hypnotic
GENERAL USES:
Insomnia
DOSAGE FORMS:
Tablets: 8 mg

RAMIPRIL
RA mi pril
TRADE NAME(S):
Altace
THERAPEUTIC CLASS:
Antihypertensive, cardiac
agent
GENERAL USES:
Hypertension, CHF
DOSAGE FORMS:
Capsules and Tablets:
1.25 mg, 2.5 mg, 5 mg,
10 mg

RAMUCIRUMAB
RA myoo SIR yoo mab
TRADE NAME(S):
Cyramza
THERAPEUTIC CLASS:
Antineoplastic
GENERAL USES:
Stomach cancer
DOSAGE FORMS:
Injection: 100 mg, 500 mg

RANIBIZUMAB
RA ni BIZ oo mab
TRADE NAME(S):
Lucentis
THERAPEUTIC CLASS:
Ocular agent

General Uses:
Wet macular degeneration,
diabetic macular edema
Dosage Forms:
Injection: 2 mL

RANITIDINE
ra NI ti deen
Trade Name(s):
Zantac 75, Zantac
EFFERdose, Zantac
GELdose
Therapeutic Class:
Gastric acid secretion
inhibitor
General Uses:
Duodenal ulcer, GERD,
heartburn (OTC)
Dosage Forms:
Tablets: 75 mg; Tablets
and Capsules: 150 mg,
300 mg; Effervescent
tablets/granules: 25 mg,
150 mg; Syrup: 15 mg/
mL; Injection: 50 mg,
150 mg, 1 g

RANOLAZINE
ra NOE la zeen
Trade Name(s):
Ranexa
Therapeutic Class:
Antianginal
General Uses:
Chronic angina
Dosage Forms:
Extended-release tablets:
500 mg

RASAGILINE
ra SA ji leen
Trade Name(s):
Azilect
Therapeutic Class:
Antiparkinson agent
General Uses:
Parkinson's disease
Dosage Forms:
Tablets: 0.5 mg, 1 mg

RASBURICASE
ras BYOOR i kayse
Trade Name(s):
Elitek
Therapeutic Class:
Antigout
General Uses:
Gout related to
chemotherapy/cancer
Dosage Forms:
Injection: 1.5 mg

RAXIBACUMAB
raks ee BAK yoo mab
Trade Name(s):
Raxibacumab
Therapeutic Class:
Antitoxin
General Uses:
Inhalation anthrax
Dosage Forms:
Injection: 1700 mg

REGADENOSON
re ga DEN oh son
Trade Name(s):
Lexiscan

THERAPEUTIC CLASS:
 Radioimaging enhancer
GENERAL USES:
 Cardiac perfusion imaging
DOSAGE FORMS:
 Injection: 0.4 mg

REGORAFENIB
REE goe RAF e nib
TRADE NAME(S):
 Stivarga
THERAPEUTIC CLASS:
 Antineoplastic
GENERAL USES:
 Metastatic colorectal
 cancer, GI stromal tumors
DOSAGE FORMS:
 Tablets: 40 mg

REPAGLINIDE
re PAG li nide
TRADE NAME(S):
 Prandin
THERAPEUTIC CLASS:
 Antidiabetic
GENERAL USES:
 Diabetes (type 2)
DOSAGE FORMS:
 Tablets: 0.5 mg, 1 mg,
 2 mg

REPAGLINIDE/ METFORMIN
re PAG li nide/met FOR min
TRADE NAME(S):
 PrandiMet
THERAPEUTIC CLASS:
 Antidiabetic

GENERAL USES:
 Diabetes (type 2)
DOSAGE FORMS:
 Tablets: 1 mg/500 mg,
 2 mg/500 mg

RETAPAMULIN
re te PAM yoo lin
TRADE NAME(S):
 Altabax
THERAPEUTIC CLASS:
 Anti-infective (topical)
GENERAL USES:
 Impetigo
DOSAGE FORMS:
 Ointment: 1%

RETEPLASE
RE ta plase
TRADE NAME(S):
 Retavase
THERAPEUTIC CLASS:
 Thrombolytic agent
GENERAL USES:
 Dissolves blood clots in
 MI
DOSAGE FORMS:
 Injection:
 10.8 international units
 (18.8 mg)

RIBAVIRIN (AEROSOL)
rye ba VYE rin
TRADE NAME(S):
 Virazole
THERAPEUTIC CLASS:
 Antiviral

GENERAL USES:
Severe lower respiratory tract infections in infants

DOSAGE FORMS:
Aerosol: 6 g

RIBAVIRIN (ORAL)
rye ba VYE rin

TRADE NAME(S):
Rebetrol

THERAPEUTIC CLASS:
Antiviral

GENERAL USES:
Chronic hepatitis C

DOSAGE FORMS:
Capsules: 200 mg

RIFABUTIN
rif a BYOO tin

TRADE NAME(S):
Mycobutin

THERAPEUTIC CLASS:
Antituberculosis agent

GENERAL USES:
Tuberculosis

DOSAGE FORMS:
Capsules: 150 mg

RIFAMPIN
rif AM pin

TRADE NAME(S):
Rifadin, Rimactane

THERAPEUTIC CLASS:
Antituberculosis agent

GENERAL USES:
Tuberculosis

DOSAGE FORMS:
Capsules: 150 mg, 300 mg; Injection: 600 mg

RIFAPENTINE
rif a PEN teen

TRADE NAME(S):
Priftin

THERAPEUTIC CLASS:
Antituberculosis agent

GENERAL USES:
Tuberculosis

DOSAGE FORMS:
Tablets: 150 mg

RIFAXIMIN
rif AKS i min

TRADE NAME(S):
Xifaxan

THERAPEUTIC CLASS:
Antibacterial

GENERAL USES:
Traveler's diarrhea, hepatic encephalopathy

DOSAGE FORMS:
Tablets: 200 mg, 550 mg

RILONACEPT
ril ON a sept

TRADE NAME(S):
Arcalyst

THERAPEUTIC CLASS:
Interleukin-1 blocker

GENERAL USES:
Cryopyrin-associated

periodic syndromes
Dosage Forms:
Injection: 160 mg

RILPIVIRINE
RIL pi VEER een
Trade Name(s):
Edurant
Therapeutic Class:
Antiviral
General Uses:
HIV infection
Dosage Forms:
Tablets: 25 mg

RILUZOLE
RIL yoo zole
Trade Name(s):
Rilutek
Therapeutic Class:
Amyotrophic lateral
sclerosis agent
General Uses:
Amyotrophic lateral
sclerosis
Dosage Forms:
Tablets: 50 mg

**RIMABOTULINUM-
TOXINB**
RYE ma BOT yoo li num
TOKS in BEE
Trade Name(s):
Myobloc
Therapeutic Class:
Toxoid
General Uses:
Cervical dystonia

Dosage Forms:
Injection: 2500 units,
5000 units, 10,000 units

RIMANTADINE
ri MAN ta deen
Trade Name(s):
Flumadine
Therapeutic Class:
Antiviral
General Uses:
Influenza A
Dosage Forms:
Tablets: 100 mg; Syrup:
50 mg/5 mL

RIMEXOLONE
ri MEKS oh lone
Trade Name(s):
Vexol
Therapeutic Class:
Ocular agent
General Uses:
Postoperative
ocular inflammation
Dosage Forms:
Ophthalmic suspension:
1%

RIOCIGUAT
RYE oh SIG yoo at
Trade Name(s):
Adempas
Therapeutic Class:
Cardiovascular agent
General Uses:
Pulmonary hypertension

DOSAGE FORMS:
Tablets: 0.5 mg, 1 mg, 1.5 mg, 2 mg, 2.5 mg

RISEDRONATE
ris ED roe nate
TRADE NAME(S):
Actonel, Atelvia
THERAPEUTIC CLASS:
Bisphosphonate
GENERAL USES:
Paget's disease, osteoporosis
DOSAGE FORMS:
Tablets: 5 mg, 30 mg, 35 mg, 75 mg, 150 mg; Extended-release tablets: 35 mg

RISPERIDONE
ris PER i done
TRADE NAME(S):
Risperdal, Risperdal Consta
THERAPEUTIC CLASS:
Antipsychotic
GENERAL USES:
Psychotic disorders
DOSAGE FORMS:
Tablets: 0.25 mg, 0.5 mg, 1 mg, 2 mg, 3 mg, 4 mg; Solution: 1 mg/mL; Injection: 25 mg, 37.5 mg, 50 mg; Orally disintegrating tablets: 0.5 mg, 1 mg, 3 mg, 4 mg

RITONAVIR
ri TOE na veer
TRADE NAME(S):
Norvir
THERAPEUTIC CLASS:
Antiviral
GENERAL USES:
HIV infection
DOSAGE FORMS:
Capsules: 100 mg; Solution: 80 mg/mL; Tablets: 100 mg

RITUXIMAB
ri TUK si mab
TRADE NAME(S):
Rituxan
THERAPEUTIC CLASS:
Monoclonal antibody
GENERAL USES:
Non-Hodgkin's lymphoma, rheumatoid arthritis
DOSAGE FORMS:
Injection: 100 mg, 500 mg

RIVAROXABAN
RIV a ROKS a ban
TRADE NAME(S):
Xarelto
THERAPEUTIC CLASS:
Anticoagulant
GENERAL USES:
Treatment and prevention of blood clots
DOSAGE FORMS:
Tablets: 10 mg, 15 mg, 20 mg

RIVASTIGMINE
ri va STIG meen
TRADE NAME(S):
Exelon
THERAPEUTIC CLASS:
Alzheimer's agent
GENERAL USES:
Alzheimer's disease and
dementia
DOSAGE FORMS:
Capsules: 1.5 mg, 3 mg,
4.5 mg, 6 mg; Solution:
2 mg/mL

**RIVASTIGMINE
(TRANSDERMAL)**
ri va STIG meen
TRADE NAME(S):
Exelon
THERAPEUTIC CLASS:
Alzheimer's agent
GENERAL USES:
Alzheimer's disease,
Parkinson's dementia
DOSAGE FORMS:
Release rate (mg/24 hr):
4.6 mg, 9.5 mg, 13.3 mg

RIZATRIPTAN
rye za TRIP tan
TRADE NAME(S):
Maxalt, Maxalt-MLT
THERAPEUTIC CLASS:
Antimigraine agent
GENERAL USES:
Migraines
DOSAGE FORMS:
Tablets and Orally

disintegrating tablets:
5 mg, 10 mg

ROFLUMILAST
roe FLOO mi last
TRADE NAME(S):
Daliresp
THERAPEUTIC CLASS:
Respiratory agent
GENERAL USES:
COPD
DOSAGE FORMS:
Tablets: 500 mcg

ROMIDEPSIN
ROE mi DEP sin
TRADE NAME(S):
Istodax
THERAPEUTIC CLASS:
Antineoplastic
GENERAL USES:
T-cell lymphoma
DOSAGE FORMS:
Injection: 10 mg

ROMIPLOSTIM
roe mi PLOE stim
TRADE NAME(S):
Nplate
THERAPEUTIC CLASS:
Hematological agent
GENERAL USES:
Thrombocytopenia
DOSAGE FORMS:
Injection: 250 mcg,
500 mcg

ROPINIROLE
roe PIN i role
TRADE NAME(S):
Requip, Requip XL
THERAPEUTIC CLASS:
Antiparkinson agent
GENERAL USES:
Parkinson's disease,
restless leg syndrome
DOSAGE FORMS:
Tablets: 0.25 mg, 0.5 mg,
1 mg, 2 mg, 5 mg;
Extended-release tablets:
2 mg, 4 mg, 6 mg, 8 mg,
12 mg

ROSIGLITAZONE
roh si GLI ta zone
TRADE NAME(S):
Avandia
THERAPEUTIC CLASS:
Antidiabetic
GENERAL USES:
Diabetes (type 2)
DOSAGE FORMS:
Tablets: 2 mg, 4 mg, 8 mg

**ROSIGLITAZONE/
GLIMEPIRIDE**
roh si GLI ta zone/GLYE me
pye ride
TRADE NAME(S):
Avandaryl
THERAPEUTIC CLASS:
Antidiabetic
GENERAL USES:
Diabetes

DOSAGE FORMS:
Tablets: 4 mg/1 mg,
4 mg/2 mg,
4 mg/4 mg

**ROSIGLITAZONE/
METFORMIN**
roh si GLI ta zone/met FOR
min
TRADE NAME(S):
Avandamet
THERAPEUTIC CLASS:
Antidiabetic
GENERAL USES:
Diabetes
DOSAGE FORMS:
Tablets: 1 mg/500 mg,
2 mg/500 mg, 4 mg/
500 mg, 2 mg/1000 mg,
4 mg/1000 mg

ROSUVASTATIN
roe soo va STAT in
TRADE NAME(S):
Crestor
THERAPEUTIC CLASS:
Antilipemic
GENERAL USES:
Hyperlipidemia
DOSAGE FORMS:
Tablets: 5 mg, 10 mg,
20 mg, 40 mg

**ROTAVIRUS LIVE
VACCINE**
ROE ta vye rus
TRADE NAME(S):
RotaTeq

THERAPEUTIC CLASS:
Vaccine

GENERAL USES:
Prevention of rotavirus gastroenteritis

DOSAGE FORMS:
Oral suspension: 2 mL

ROTIGOTINE (TRANSDERMAL)
roe TIG oh tine

TRADE NAME(S):
Neupro

THERAPEUTIC CLASS:
Antiparkinson agent

GENERAL USES:
Parkinson's disease, restless leg syndrome

DOSAGE FORMS:
Patch: 1 mg, 2 mg, 3 mg, 4 mg, 6 mg, 8 mg

RUFINAMIDE
roo FIN a mide

TRADE NAME(S):
Banzel

THERAPEUTIC CLASS:
Anticonvulsant

GENERAL USES:
Seizures

DOSAGE FORMS:
Tablets: 200 mg, 400 mg; Suspension (oral): 40 mg/mL

RUXOLITINIB
RUX oh LI ti nib

TRADE NAME(S):
Jakafi

THERAPEUTIC CLASS:
Kinase inhibitor

GENERAL USES:
Myelofibrosis

DOSAGE FORMS:
Tablets: 5 mg, 10 mg, 15 mg, 20 mg, 25 mg

SACROSIDASE
sak ROE si dase

TRADE NAME(S):
Sucraid

THERAPEUTIC CLASS:
Enzyme replacement

GENERAL USES:
Sucrase-isomaltase deficiency

DOSAGE FORMS:
Solution: 8500 international units/ mL

SALMETEROL
sal ME te role

TRADE NAME(S):
Serevent, Serevent Diskus

THERAPEUTIC CLASS:
Bronchodilator

GENERAL USES:
Asthma, COPD, bronchospasm

DOSAGE FORMS:
Aerosol: 25 mcg/

actuation; Inhalation
powder pack:
50 mcg

SALSALATE
SAL sa late
TRADE NAME(S):
Disalcid, Amigesic,
Salsitab
THERAPEUTIC CLASS:
Anti-inflammatory/
analgesic
GENERAL USES:
Pain, osteoarthritis,
rheumatoid arthritis
DOSAGE FORMS:
Capsules: 500 mg;
Tablets: 500 mg, 750 mg

SAPROPTERIN
sap roe TER in
TRADE NAME(S):
Kuvan
THERAPEUTIC CLASS:
Enzyme
GENERAL USES:
Reduce blood
phenylalanine
DOSAGE FORMS:
Tablets: 100 mg;
Solution: 100 mg

SAQUINAVIR
sa KWIN a veer
TRADE NAME(S):
Invirase
THERAPEUTIC CLASS:
Antiviral

GENERAL USES:
HIV infection
DOSAGE FORMS:
Tablets: 200 mg, 500 mg

SAXAGLIPTIN
SAX a GLIP tin
TRADE NAME(S):
Onglyza
THERAPEUTIC CLASS:
Antidiabetic
GENERAL USES:
Diabetes (type 2)
DOSAGE FORMS:
Tablets: 2.5 mg, 5 mg

SCOPOLAMINE
skoe POL a meen
TRADE NAME(S):
Transderm-Scop
THERAPEUTIC CLASS:
Antiemetic/antivertigo
agent
GENERAL USES:
Motion sickness
DOSAGE FORMS:
Transdermal patch:
1.5 mg

SECOBARBITAL
see koe BAR bi tal
TRADE NAME(S):
Seconal
THERAPEUTIC CLASS:
Sedative/hypnotic
GENERAL USES:
Insomnia (short-term
therapy)

DOSAGE FORMS:
Capsules: 100 mg

SECRETIN
se KREE tin
TRADE NAME(S):
SecreFlo
THERAPEUTIC CLASS:
Diagnostic agent
GENERAL USES:
Pancreatic dysfunction/
tumor
DOSAGE FORMS:
Injection: 16 mcg

SELEGILINE
se LE ji leen
TRADE NAME(S):
Eldepryl, Zelapar
THERAPEUTIC CLASS:
Antiparkinson agent
GENERAL USES:
Parkinson's disease
DOSAGE FORMS:
Tablets and Capsules:
5 mg; Orally disintegrating
tablets: 1.25 mg

SELEGILINE
(TRANSDERMAL)
se LE ji leen
TRADE NAME(S):
Emsam
THERAPEUTIC CLASS:
CNS agent,
antidepressant
GENERAL USES:
Depression

DOSAGE FORMS:
Patch: 6 mg, 9 mg,
12 mg

SERTACONAZOLE
(TOPICAL)
ser ta KOE na zole
TRADE NAME(S):
Ertaczo
THERAPEUTIC CLASS:
Antifungal
GENERAL USES:
Tinea pedis
DOSAGE FORMS:
Cream: 2%

SERTRALINE
SER tra leen
TRADE NAME(S):
Zoloft
THERAPEUTIC CLASS:
Antidepressant
GENERAL USES:
Depression, OCD, panic
disorder, social anxiety,
PMDD
DOSAGE FORMS:
Tablets: 25 mg, 50 mg,
100 mg; Concentrated
solution: 20 mg/mL

SEVELAMER
CARBONATE
se VEL a mer
TRADE NAME(S):
Renvela
THERAPEUTIC CLASS:
Phosphate-binding agent

GENERAL USES:
High phosphorus levels in kidney disease

DOSAGE FORMS:
Suspension (oral): 800 mg, 2.4 g; Tablets: 800 mg

SEVELAMER HCL
se VEL a mer

TRADE NAME(S):
Renagel

THERAPEUTIC CLASS:
Phosphate-binding agent

GENERAL USES:
High phosphorus levels in kidney disease

DOSAGE FORMS:
Tablets: 400 mg, 800 mg

SILDENAFIL
sil DEN a fil

TRADE NAME(S):
Viagra

THERAPEUTIC CLASS:
Impotence agent

GENERAL USES:
Erectile dysfunction

DOSAGE FORMS:
Tablets: 25 mg, 50 mg, 100 mg

SILDENAFIL CITRATE
sil DEN a fil

TRADE NAME(S):
Revatio

THERAPEUTIC CLASS:
Antihypertensive

GENERAL USES:
PAH

DOSAGE FORMS:
Injection: 10 mg; Suspension (oral): 10 mg/mL; Tablets: 20 mg

SILODOSIN
sil OH doe sin

TRADE NAME(S):
Rapaflo

THERAPEUTIC CLASS:
BPH agent

GENERAL USES:
BPH

DOSAGE FORMS:
Capsules: 4 mg, 8 mg

SILTUXIMAB
sil TUX i mab

TRADE NAME(S):
Sylvant

THERAPEUTIC CLASS:
Antibody

GENERAL USES:
Multicentric Castleman's disease

DOSAGE FORMS:
Injection: 100 mg, 400 mg

SIMEPREVIR
sim E pre veer

TRADE NAME(S):
Olysio

THERAPEUTIC CLASS:
Antiviral

GENERAL USES:
Hepatitis C virus
DOSAGE FORMS:
Capsules: 150 mg

SIMVASTATIN
SIM va stat in
TRADE NAME(S):
Zocor
THERAPEUTIC CLASS:
Antilipemic
GENERAL USES:
Hyperlipidemia, CHD
DOSAGE FORMS:
Tablets: 5 mg, 10 mg,
20 mg, 40 mg, 80 mg

SIMVASTATIN/NIACIN
SIM va stat in/NYE a sin
TRADE NAME(S):
Simcor
THERAPEUTIC CLASS:
Antilipemic
GENERAL USES:
Hyperlipidemia
DOSAGE FORMS:
Extended-release tablets:
20 mg/500 mg, 20 mg/
750 mg, 20 mg/1000 mg

SINECATECHINS (TOPICAL)
sin a CAT ah kins
TRADE NAME(S):
Veregen
THERAPEUTIC CLASS:
Dermatologic agent

GENERAL USES:
Genital and perianal warts
DOSAGE FORMS:
Ointment: 15%

SIROLIMUS
sir OH li mus
TRADE NAME(S):
Rapamune
THERAPEUTIC CLASS:
Immunomodulator
GENERAL USES:
Prevent organ transplant
rejection
DOSAGE FORMS:
Solution: 1 mg/mL;
Tablets: 1 mg

SITAGLIPTIN
sit a GLIP tin
TRADE NAME(S):
Januvia
THERAPEUTIC CLASS:
Antidiabetic
GENERAL USES:
Diabetes
DOSAGE FORMS:
Tablets: 25 mg, 50 mg,
100 mg

SITAGLIPTIN/ METFORMIN
sit a GLIP tin/met FOR min
TRADE NAME(S):
Janumet, Janumet XR
THERAPEUTIC CLASS:
Antidiabetic

GENERAL USES:
  Diabetes (type 2)
DOSAGE FORMS:
  Extended-release tablets
  and Tablets: 50 mg/500
  mg, 50 mg/1000 mg;
  Extended-release
  tablets: 100 mg/1000 mg

SODIUM PICOSULFATE/ MAGNESIUM OXIDE/ CITRIC ACID

SOE dee um PI koe SUL fate/
mag NEE zhum OKS ide/
SI trik AS id
TRADE NAME(S):
  Prepopik
THERAPEUTIC CLASS:
  Gastrointestinal agent
GENERAL USES:
  Laxative for colonoscopy
DOSAGE FORMS:
  Oral solution (sachet):
  10 mg/3.5 mg/12 mg

SODIUM SULFATE/ POTASSIUM SULFATE/ MAGNESIUM SULFATE

SOE dee um SUL fate/ poe
TASS ee um SUL fate/ mag
NEE zhum SUL fate
TRADE NAME(S):
  Suprep
THERAPEUTIC CLASS:
  Laxative
GENERAL USES:
  Bowel evacuation

DOSAGE FORMS:
  Solution (oral): 6 oz

SODIUM TETRADECYL SULFATE

SO dee um tetra DEK il
TRADE NAME(S):
  Sotradecol
THERAPEUTIC CLASS:
  Sclerosing agent
GENERAL USES:
  Varicose veins
DOSAGE FORMS:
  Injection: 1%, 3%

SOFOSBUVIR

soe FOS byoo veer
TRADE NAME(S):
  Sovaldi
THERAPEUTIC CLASS:
  Antiviral
GENERAL USES:
  Hepatitis C virus
DOSAGE FORMS:
  Tablets: 400 mg

SOLIFENACIN SUCCINATE

sol i FEN a sin
TRADE NAME(S):
  VESIcare
THERAPEUTIC CLASS:
  Anticholinerigc
GENERAL USES:
  Overactive bladder
DOSAGE FORMS:
  Tablets: 5 mg, 10 mg

SORAFENIB TOSYLATE
sor AF e nib TOE sil ate
Trade Name(s):
Nexavar
Therapeutic Class:
Antineoplastic
General Uses:
Advanced renal cell carcinoma, thyroid cancer, hepatocellular carcinoma
Dosage Forms:
Tablets: 200 mg

SOTALOL
SOE ta lole
Trade Name(s):
Betapace, Betapace AF, Sotalol, Sotylize
Therapeutic Class:
Antiarrhythmic
General Uses:
Arrhythmias
Dosage Forms:
Injection: 150 mg; Tablets: 80 mg, 120 mg, 160 mg, 240 mg; Oral solution: 5 mg/mL

SPARFLOXACIN
spar FLOKS a sin
Trade Name(s):
Zagam
Therapeutic Class:
Anti-infective
General Uses:
Bacterial infections
Dosage Forms:
Tablets: 200 mg

SPINOSAD
SPIN oh sad
Trade Name(s):
Natroba
Therapeutic Class:
Pediculicide
General Uses:
Head lice
Dosage Forms:
Suspension (topical): 0.9%

SPIRONOLACTONE
speer on oh LAK tone
Trade Name(s):
Aldactone
Therapeutic Class:
Diuretic
General Uses:
Edema, hypertension, hyperaldosteronism
Dosage Forms:
Tablets: 25 mg, 50 mg, 100 mg

STAVUDINE (d4T)
STAV yoo deen
Trade Name(s):
Zerit
Therapeutic Class:
Antiviral
General Uses:
HIV infection
Dosage Forms:
Capsules: 15 mg, 20 mg, 30 mg, 40 mg; Powder: 1 mg/mL

STREPTOKINASE
strep toe KYE nase
TRADE NAME(S):
 Streptase
THERAPEUTIC CLASS:
 Thrombolytic agent
GENERAL USES:
 Dissolves blood
 clots
DOSAGE FORMS:
 Injection: 250,000
 international units,
 750,000 international
 units, 1.5 million
 international units

SUCCIMER
SUCK sih mer
TRADE NAME(S):
 Chemet
THERAPEUTIC CLASS:
 Heavy metal binder
GENERAL USES:
 Lead poisoning
DOSAGE FORMS:
 Capsules: 100 mg

SUCRALFATE
soo KRAL fate
TRADE NAME(S):
 Carafate
THERAPEUTIC CLASS:
 Gastric protectant
GENERAL USES:
 Duodenal ulcer
DOSAGE FORMS:
 Tablets: 1 g; Suspension:
 1 g/10 mL

SUCROFERRIC OXYHYDROXIDE
soo kroe FER ik oks ee hye DROKS ide
TRADE NAME(S):
 Velphoro
THERAPEUTIC CLASS:
 Phosphate binder
GENERAL USES:
 Elevated phosphorous
 levels
DOSAGE FORMS:
 Chewable tablets: 500 mg

SULFADIAZINE
sul fa DYE a zeen
TRADE NAME(S):
 Microsulfon
THERAPEUTIC CLASS:
 Anti-infective
GENERAL USES:
 Bacterial infections
DOSAGE FORMS:
 Tablets: 500 mg

SULFASALAZINE
sul fa SAL a zeen
TRADE NAME(S):
 Azulfidine, Azulfidine EN
THERAPEUTIC CLASS:
 GI agent
GENERAL USES:
 Ulcerative colitis,
 rheumatoid arthritis
DOSAGE FORMS:
 Tablets: 500 mg;
 Delayed-release
 tablets: 500 mg

SULFINPYRAZONE
sul fin PEER a zone
Trade Name(s):
Anturane
Therapeutic Class:
Gout agent
General Uses:
Gouty arthritis
Dosage Forms:
Tablets: 100 mg;
Capsules: 200 mg

SULINDAC
sul IN dak
Trade Name(s):
Clinoril
Therapeutic Class:
Anti-inflammatory/
analgesic
General Uses:
Various arthritis
conditions, pain
Dosage Forms:
Tablets: 150 mg, 200 mg

SUMATRIPTAN
soo ma TRIP tan
Trade Name(s):
Alsuma, Imitrex, Sumavel
Dosepro, Zecuity
Therapeutic Class:
Antimigraine
General Uses:
Migraines
Dosage Forms:
Tablets: 25 mg, 50 mg,
100 mg; Nasal spray:
5 mg, 20 mg; Injection:
6 mg; Transdermal
system: 6.5 mg

**SUMATRIPTAN/
NAPROXEN**
soo ma TRIP tan/na PROKS
en
Trade Name(s):
Treximet
Therapeutic Class:
Antimigraine/NSAID
General Uses:
Migraines
Dosage Forms:
Tablets: 85 mg/500 mg

SUNITINIB MALEATE
su NIT i nib
Trade Name(s):
Sutent
Therapeutic Class:
Antineoplastic
General Uses:
Gastric and renal cancer
Dosage Forms:
Capsules: 12.5 mg,
25 mg, 50 mg

SUPROFEN
soo PRO fen
Trade Name(s):
Profenal
Therapeutic Class:
Ocular agent
General Uses:
Maintain pupil dilation
during surgery

DOSAGE FORMS:
Ophthalmic solution: 1%

SUVOREXANT
soo voh REKS ant
TRADE NAME(S):
Belsomra
THERAPEUTIC CLASS:
Sedative, hypnotic
GENERAL USES:
Insomnia
DOSAGE FORMS:
Tablets: 5 mg, 10 mg, 15 mg, 20 mg

TACRINE
TAK reen
TRADE NAME(S):
Cognex
THERAPEUTIC CLASS:
Alzheimer's agent
GENERAL USES:
Alzheimer's disease
DOSAGE FORMS:
Capsules: 10 mg, 20 mg, 30 mg, 40 mg

TACROLIMUS
ta KROE li mus
TRADE NAME(S):
Astragraf XL, Prograf
THERAPEUTIC CLASS:
Immunosuppressant
GENERAL USES:
Prevent organ transplant rejection
DOSAGE FORMS:
Capsules: 1 mg, 5 mg; Extended-release capsules: 0.5 mg, 1 mg, 5 mg

TADALAFIL
tah DA la fil
TRADE NAME(S):
Adcirca, Cialis
THERAPEUTIC CLASS:
Impotence agent, antihypertensive
GENERAL USES:
Erectile dysfunction, PAH, BPH
DOSAGE FORMS:
Tablets: 5 mg, 10 mg, 20 mg

TAFLUPROST
TA floo prost
TRADE NAME(S):
Zioptan
THERAPEUTIC CLASS:
Ocular agent
GENERAL USES:
Glaucoma/ocular hypertension
DOSAGE FORMS:
Ophthalmic solution: 0.0015%

TALIGLUCERASE ALFA
TAL i GLOO ser ase AL fa
TRADE NAME(S):
Elelyso

THERAPEUTIC CLASS:
Enzyme replacement
GENERAL USES:
Type 1 Gaucher's disease
DOSAGE FORMS:
Injection: 200 units

TAMOXIFEN
ta MOKS i fen
TRADE NAME(S):
Nolvadex, Soltamox
THERAPEUTIC CLASS:
Antiestrogen/
antineoplastic
GENERAL USES:
Breast cancer
DOSAGE FORMS:
Tablets: 10 mg, 20 mg;
Solution: 10 mg/5 mL

TAMSULOSIN
tam SOO loe sin
TRADE NAME(S):
Flomax
THERAPEUTIC CLASS:
Urologic agent
GENERAL USES:
BPH
DOSAGE FORMS:
Capsules: 0.4 mg

TAPENTADOL HCL
ta PEN ta dol
TRADE NAME(S):
Nucynta
THERAPEUTIC CLASS:
Analgesic (narcotic)

GENERAL USES:
Pain
DOSAGE FORMS:
Tablets: 50 mg, 75 mg,
100 mg; Solution: 20 mg/
mL

TASIMELTEON
TAS i MEL tee on
TRADE NAME(S):
Hetlioz
THERAPEUTIC CLASS:
Sedative/hypnotic
GENERAL USES:
Insomnia
DOSAGE FORMS:
Capsules: 20 mg

TAVABOROLE
ta va BOR ole
TRADE NAME(S):
Kerydin
THERAPEUTIC CLASS:
Antifungal
GENERAL USES:
Toenail fungal infection
DOSAGE FORMS:
Solution: 5%

TAZAROTENE
taz AR oh teen
TRADE NAME(S):
Tazorac, Fabior
THERAPEUTIC CLASS:
Retinoid (topical)
GENERAL USES:
Acne, psoriasis

DOSAGE FORMS:
Gel: 0.05%, 0.1%;
Foam: 0.1%

TBO-FILGRASTIM
TEE boe fil GRA stim
TRADE NAME(S):
Granix
THERAPEUTIC CLASS:
Hematological agent
GENERAL USES:
Malignancy-related
neutropenia
DOSAGE FORMS:
Injection: 300 mcg,
480 mcg

TEDIZOLID PHOSPHATE
ted A zol id
TRADE NAME(S):
Sivextro
THERAPEUTIC CLASS:
Anti-infective
GENERAL USES:
Bacterial infections
DOSAGE FORMS:
Injection: 200 mg;
Tablets: 200 mg

TEDUGLUTIDE
te DOOG lu tide
TRADE NAME(S):
Gattex
THERAPEUTIC CLASS:
GI agent
GENERAL USES:
Short bowel syndrome

DOSAGE FORMS:
Injection: 5 mg

TELAPREVIR
tel A pre veer
TRADE NAME(S):
Incivek
THERAPEUTIC CLASS:
Antiviral
GENERAL USES:
Chronic hepatitis C
DOSAGE FORMS:
Tablets: 375 mg

TELAVANCIN
TEL a VAN sin
TRADE NAME(S):
Vibativ
THERAPEUTIC CLASS:
Anti-infective
GENERAL USES:
Bacterial infections
DOSAGE FORMS:
Injection: 250 mg, 750 mg

TELBIVUDINE
tel BI vyoo deen
TRADE NAME(S):
Tyzeka
THERAPEUTIC CLASS:
Antiviral
GENERAL USES:
Hepatitis B
DOSAGE FORMS:
Oral solution: 100 mg/
5 mL; Tablets: 600 mg

TELITHROMYCIN
tel ITH roe my sin
TRADE NAME(S):
Ketek
THERAPEUTIC CLASS:
Anti-infective
GENERAL USES:
Community-acquired
pneumonia, acute
bronchitis/sinusitis
DOSAGE FORMS:
Tablets: 400 mg

TELMISARTAN
tel mi SAR tan
TRADE NAME(S):
Micardis
THERAPEUTIC CLASS:
Antihypertensive
GENERAL USES:
Hypertension
DOSAGE FORMS:
Tablets: 40 mg, 80 mg

TELMISARTAN/HCTZ
tel mi SAR tan/hye droe klor
oh THYE a zide
TRADE NAME(S):
Micardis HCT
THERAPEUTIC CLASS:
Antihypertensive/diuretic
GENERAL USES:
Hypertension
DOSAGE FORMS:
Tablets: 40 mg/12.5 mg,
80 mg/12.5 mg, 80 mg/
25 mg

TEMAZEPAM
te MAZ e pam
TRADE NAME(S):
Restoril
THERAPEUTIC CLASS:
Sedative/hypnotic
GENERAL USES:
Insomnia
DOSAGE FORMS:
Capsules: 7.5 mg, 15 mg,
30 mg

TEMOZOLOMIDE
te moe ZOE loe mide
TRADE NAME(S):
Temodar
THERAPEUTIC CLASS:
Antineoplastic
GENERAL USES:
Astrocytoma (brain tumor)
DOSAGE FORMS:
Capsules: 5 mg, 20 mg,
100 mg, 250 mg;
Injection: 100 mg

TEMSIROLIMUS
tem sir OH li mus
TRADE NAME(S):
Torisel
THERAPEUTIC CLASS:
Antineoplastic
GENERAL USES:
Kidney cancer
DOSAGE FORMS:
Injection: 25 mg

TENECTEPLASE
ten EK te plase
TRADE NAME(S):
TNKase
THERAPEUTIC CLASS:
Thrombolytic
GENERAL USES:
Dissolves blood clots in MI
DOSAGE FORMS:
Injection: 50 mg

TENOFOVIR
te NOE fo veer
TRADE NAME(S):
Viread
THERAPEUTIC CLASS:
Antiviral
GENERAL USES:
HIV infection
DOSAGE FORMS:
Tablets: 150 mg, 200 mg,
250 mg, 300 mg; Powder
(oral): 40 mg

**TENOFOVIR/
EMTRICITABINE**
te NOE fo veer/em trye SYE
ta been
TRADE NAME(S):
Truvada
THERAPEUTIC CLASS:
Antiviral
GENERAL USES:
HIV infection
DOSAGE FORMS:
Tablets: 300 mg/200 mg

TERAZOSIN
ter AY zoe sin
TRADE NAME(S):
Terazosin
THERAPEUTIC CLASS:
Antihypertensive, BPH
agent
GENERAL USES:
Hypertension, BPH
DOSAGE FORMS:
Capsules, Tablets: 1 mg,
2 mg, 5 mg, 10 mg

TERBINAFINE
TER bin a feen
TRADE NAME(S):
Lamisil
THERAPEUTIC CLASS:
Antifungal
GENERAL USES:
Nail fungal infections,
ringworm, athlete's foot
DOSAGE FORMS:
Tablets: 250 mg; Cream
and Gel: 1%

TERBUTALINE
ter BYOO ta leen
TRADE NAME(S):
Brethine
THERAPEUTIC CLASS:
Bronchodilator
GENERAL USES:
Bronchospasm, asthma
DOSAGE FORMS:
Tablets: 2.5 mg, 5 mg;
Inhaler: 0.2 mg/inhalation;
Injection: 1 mg

TERCONAZOLE
ter KONE a zole
TRADE NAME(S):
Terazol-7, Terazol-3
THERAPEUTIC CLASS:
Vaginal antifungal
GENERAL USES:
Vaginal candidiasis
DOSAGE FORMS:
Vaginal cream:
0.4%, 0.8%; Vaginal
suppository: 80 mg

TERIFLUNOMIDE
ter i FLOO no mide
TRADE NAME(S):
Aubagio
THERAPEUTIC CLASS:
Multiple sclerosis agent
GENERAL USES:
Multiple sclerosis
DOSAGE FORMS:
Tablets: 7 mg, 14 mg

TERIPARATIDE
ter i PAR a tide
TRADE NAME(S):
Forteo
THERAPEUTIC CLASS:
Parathyroid hormone
GENERAL USES:
Post menopausal
osteoporosis
DOSAGE FORMS:
Injection: 750 mcg

TESAMORELIN
TES a moe REL in
TRADE NAME(S):
Egrifta
THERAPEUTIC CLASS:
Hormone
GENERAL USES:
HIV lipodystrophy
DOSAGE FORMS:
Injection: 1 mg

**TESTOSTERONE
(BUCCAL)**
tes TOS ter one
TRADE NAME(S):
Striant
THERAPEUTIC CLASS:
Hormone (testosterone)
GENERAL USES:
Testosterone replacement
DOSAGE FORMS:
Buccal system: 30 mg

**TESTOSTERONE
(INTRANASAL)**
tes TOS ter one
TRADE NAME(S):
Natesto
THERAPEUTIC CLASS:
Hormone
GENERAL USES:
Replacement therapy in
men
DOSAGE FORMS:
Nasal gel: 5.5 mg/pump

TESTOSTERONE (TOPICAL)
tes TOS ter one
TRADE NAME(S):
Androgel, Axiron, Fortesta, Testim, Vogelxo
THERAPEUTIC CLASS:
Hormone (testosterone)
GENERAL USES:
Replacement therapy in men
DOSAGE FORMS:
Gel: 1%, 1.6%, 12.5 mg, 50 mg; Spray: 30 mg/ spray

TESTOSTERONE (TRANSDERMAL)
tes TOS ter one
TRADE NAME(S):
Androderm
THERAPEUTIC CLASS:
Hormone
GENERAL USES:
Replacement therapy in men
DOSAGE FORMS:
Patch: 2.5 mg/24 hr, 5 mg/24 hr

TESTOSTERONE UNDECANOATE
tes TOS ter one
TRADE NAME(S):
Aveed
THERAPEUTIC CLASS:
Hormone

GENERAL USES:
Replacement therapy in men
DOSAGE FORMS:
Injection: 750 mg

TETRABENAZINE
tet ra BEN a zeen
TRADE NAME(S):
Xenazine
THERAPEUTIC CLASS:
Monoamine depletor
GENERAL USES:
Chorea in Huntington's disease
DOSAGE FORMS:
Tablets: 12.5 mg, 25 mg

TETRACYCLINE
tet ra SYE kleen
TRADE NAME(S):
Sumycin, Tetracyn
THERAPEUTIC CLASS:
Anti-infective
GENERAL USES:
Bacterial infections
DOSAGE FORMS:
Capsules and Tablets: 250 mg, 500 mg; Suspension: 125 mg/ 5 mL

THALIDOMIDE
tha LI doe mide
TRADE NAME(S):
Thalomid
THERAPEUTIC CLASS:
Immunomodulator

GENERAL USES:
Erythema nodosum
leprosum (skin disorder),
multiple myeloma

DOSAGE FORMS:
Capsules: 50 mg, 100 mg,
200 mg

THEOPHYLLINE
thee OFF i lin

TRADE NAME(S):
Slo-Phyllin, Theo-Dur,
several others

THERAPEUTIC CLASS:
Bronchodilator

GENERAL USES:
Bronchial asthma,
bronchospasm

DOSAGE FORMS:
Tablets: 100 mg, 125 mg,
200 mg, 250 mg, 300 mg;
Capsules: 100 mg,
200 mg; Syrup and
Elixir: 26.7 mg/5 mL;
Syrup: 50 mg/5 mL;
Timed-release tablets and
capsules: 50 mg, 75 mg,
100 mg, 125 mg, 200 mg,
250 mg, 300 mg, 400 mg,
500 mg, 600 mg

THIORIDAZINE
thye oh RID a zeen

TRADE NAME(S):
Mellaril, Mellaril-S

THERAPEUTIC CLASS:
Antipsychotic

GENERAL USES:
Psychotic disorders,
emesis

DOSAGE FORMS:
Tablets: 10 mg, 15 mg,
25 mg, 50 mg, 100 mg,
150 mg, 200 mg;
Concentrated solution:
30 mg/mL, 100 mg/mL;
Suspension: 25 mg/5 mL,
100 mg/5 mL

THIOTHIXENE
thye oh THIKS een

TRADE NAME(S):
Navane

THERAPEUTIC CLASS:
Antipsychotic

GENERAL USES:
Psychotic/behavioral
disorders

DOSAGE FORMS:
Capsules: 1 mg, 2 mg,
5 mg, 10 mg, 20 mg;
Concentrated solution:
5 mg/mL

THYROID DESICCATED
THYE roid DESS i kate ed

TRADE NAME(S):
Armour-Thyroid, Nature-
Throid, Westhroid,
Biothroid

THERAPEUTIC CLASS:
Hormone

GENERAL USES:
Hypothyroidism

DOSAGE FORMS:
  Tablets: 15 mg, 30 mg,
  32.4 mg, 32.5 mg,
  60 mg, 64.8 mg,
  65 mg, 90 mg, 120 mg,
  129.6 mg, 130 mg,
  180 mg, 194.4 mg,
  195 mg, 240 mg, 300 mg;
  Capsules: 7.5 mg, 15 mg,
  30 mg, 60 mg, 90 mg,
  120 mg, 150 mg, 180 mg,
  240 mg

TIAGABINE
tye AG a been
TRADE NAME(S):
  Gabitril
THERAPEUTIC CLASS:
  Anticonvulsant
GENERAL USES:
  Seizures
DOSAGE FORMS:
  Tablets: 4 mg, 12 mg,
  16 mg, 20 mg

TICAGRELOR
tye KA grel or
TRADE NAME(S):
  Brilinta
THERAPEUTIC CLASS:
  Anticoagulant
GENERAL USES:
  Preventive therapy for
  blood clots
DOSAGE FORMS:
  Tablets: 90 mg

TICARCILLIN
tye kar SIL in
TRADE NAME(S):
  Ticar
THERAPEUTIC CLASS:
  Anti-infective
GENERAL USES:
  Bacterial infections
DOSAGE FORMS:
  Injection: 1 g, 3 g, 6 g,
  20 g, 30 g

TICARCILLIN/ CLAVULANATE POTASSIUM
tye kar SIL in/klav yoo LAN
ate
TRADE NAME(S):
  Timentin
THERAPEUTIC CLASS:
  Anti-infective
GENERAL USES:
  Bacterial infections
DOSAGE FORMS:
  Injection: 3 g/0.1 g

TICLOPIDINE
tye KLOE pi deen
TRADE NAME(S):
  Ticlid
THERAPEUTIC CLASS:
  Antiplatelet agent
GENERAL USES:
  Reduce risk of stroke due
  to clots
DOSAGE FORMS:
  Tablets: 250 mg

TIGECYCLINE
ty ge SYE kleen
TRADE NAME(S):
  Tygacil
THERAPEUTIC CLASS:
  Anti-infective
GENERAL USES:
  Various infections
DOSAGE FORMS:
  Injection: 50 mg

TILUDRONATE
tye LOO droe nate
TRADE NAME(S):
  Skelid
THERAPEUTIC CLASS:
  Bisphosphonate
GENERAL USES:
  Paget's disease
DOSAGE FORMS:
  Tablets: 240 mg

TIMOLOL (OCULAR)
TYE moe lole
TRADE NAME(S):
  Betimol, Timoptic, Istalol
THERAPEUTIC CLASS:
  Ocular agent
GENERAL USES:
  Glaucoma/ocular
  hypertension
DOSAGE FORMS:
  Ophthalmic solution:
  0.25%, 0.5%

TIMOLOL (ORAL)
TYE moe lole
TRADE NAME(S):
  Blocadren
THERAPEUTIC CLASS:
  Antihypertensive, cardiac
  agent, anti-migraine agent
GENERAL USES:
  Hypertension, MI,
  migraines
DOSAGE FORMS:
  Tablets: 5 mg, 10 mg,
  20 mg

TIMOLOL/HCTZ
TYE moe lole/hye droe klor
oh THYE a zide
TRADE NAME(S):
  Timolide
THERAPEUTIC CLASS:
  Antihypertensive/
  diuretic
GENERAL USES:
  Hypertension
DOSAGE FORMS:
  Tablets: 10 mg/25 mg

TINIDAZOLE
ty NI da zole
TRADE NAME(S):
  Tindamax
THERAPEUTIC CLASS:
  Antifungal
GENERAL USES:
  Antiprotozoal
DOSAGE FORMS:
  Tablets: 250 mg, 500 mg

TIOTROPIUM
ty oh TROE pee um
TRADE NAME(S):
Spiriva Respimat, Spiriva
THERAPEUTIC CLASS:
Bronchodilator
GENERAL USES:
COPD
DOSAGE FORMS:
Inhaler capsules: 18 mcg;
Inhalation: 2.5 mcg/
actuation

TIPRANAVIR
tip RA na veer
TRADE NAME(S):
Aptivus
THERAPEUTIC CLASS:
Antiviral
GENERAL USES:
HIV infection
DOSAGE FORMS:
Capsules: 250 mg; Oral
solution: 100 mg/mL

TIZANIDINE
tye ZAN i deen
TRADE NAME(S):
Zanaflex
THERAPEUTIC CLASS:
Skeletal muscle relaxant
GENERAL USES:
Muscle spasticity
DOSAGE FORMS:
Tablets: 4 mg

TOBRAMYCIN (OCULAR)
toe bra MYE sin
TRADE NAME(S):
Tobrex, AKTob
THERAPEUTIC CLASS:
Ocular agent
(anti-infective)
GENERAL USES:
Ocular infections
DOSAGE FORMS:
Ophthalmic solution:
0.3%; Ophthalmic
ointment: 3 mg/g

TOBRAMYCIN SULFATE
toe bra MYE sin
TRADE NAME(S):
Nebcin, Bethkig, Tob,
Podhaler
THERAPEUTIC CLASS:
Anti-infective
GENERAL USES:
Bacterial infections
DOSAGE FORMS:
Injection: 20 mg, 60 mg,
80 mg, 1.2 g; Nebulizer
solution: 300 mg;
Inhalation: 28 mg

TOBRAMYCIN/
DEXAMETHASONE
(OCULAR)
toe bra MYE sin/deks a
METH a sone
TRADE NAME(S):
TobraDex, TobraDex ST
THERAPEUTIC CLASS:
Anti-infective/

anti-inflammatory
(ocular)

GENERAL USES:
Ocular infection/
inflammation

DOSAGE FORMS:
Ophthalmic
suspension: 0.05%/0.3%,
0.3%/0.1%;
Ophthalmic ointment:
0.3%/0.1%

TOCAINIDE
toe KAY nide

TRADE NAME(S):
Tonocard

THERAPEUTIC CLASS:
Antiarrhythmic

GENERAL USES:
Ventricular arrhythmias

DOSAGE FORMS:
Tablets: 400 mg, 600 mg

TOCILIZUMAB
TOE si LIZ oo mab

TRADE NAME(S):
Actemra

THERAPEUTIC CLASS:
Interleukin inhibitor

GENERAL USES:
Rheumatoid arthritis,
juvenile idiopathic arthritis

DOSAGE FORMS:
Injection: 80 mg, 200 mg,
400 mg, 162 mg

TOFACITINIB
TOE fa SYE ti nib

TRADE NAME(S):
Xeljanz

THERAPEUTIC CLASS:
Antirheumatic agent

GENERAL USES:
Rheumatoid arthritis

DOSAGE FORMS:
Tablets: 5 mg

TOLAZAMIDE
tole AZ a mide

TRADE NAME(S):
Tolinase

THERAPEUTIC CLASS:
Antidiabetic

GENERAL USES:
Diabetes (type 2)

DOSAGE FORMS:
Tablets: 100 mg, 250 mg,
500 mg

TOLBUTAMIDE
tole BYOO ta mide

TRADE NAME(S):
Orinase

THERAPEUTIC CLASS:
Antidiabetic

GENERAL USES:
Diabetes (type 2)

DOSAGE FORMS:
Tablets: 500 mg

TOLCAPONE
TOLE ka pone

TRADE NAME(S):
Tasmar

Therapeutic Class:
  Antiparkinson agent
General Uses:
  Parkinson's
  disease
Dosage Forms:
  Tablets: 100 mg, 200 mg

TOLMETIN
TOLE met in
Trade Name(s):
  Tolectin
Therapeutic Class:
  Anti-inflammatory/
  analgesic
General Uses:
  Osteoarthritis, rheumatoid
  arthritis
Dosage Forms:
  Tablets: 200 mg, 600 mg;
  Capsules: 400 mg

TOLTERODINE
tole TER oh deen
Trade Name(s):
  Detrol, Detrol LA
Therapeutic Class:
  Antispasmodic
General Uses:
  Bladder instability
Dosage Forms:
  Tablets: 1 mg, 2 mg;
  Extended-release
  capsules: 2 mg, 4 mg

TOLVAPTAN
tol VAP tan
Trade Name(s):
  Samsca
Therapeutic Class:
  Vasopressin receptor
  antagonist
General Uses:
  Hypervolemic and
  euvolemic hyponatremia
Dosage Forms:
  Tablets: 15 mg, 30 mg,
  60 mg

TOPIRAMATE
toe PYRE a mate
Trade Name(s):
  Quaexy XR, Topamax,
  Trokendi XR
Therapeutic Class:
  Anticonvulsant
General Uses:
  Seizures, migraines
Dosage Forms:
  Extended-release
  capsules: 25 mg, 50 mg,
  100 mg, 150 mg, 200 mg;
  Tablets: 25 mg, 100 mg,
  200 mg; Sprinkle
  capsules: 15 mg, 25 mg

TOPOTECAN HCL
toe poe TEE kan
Trade Name(s):
  Hycamtin
Therapeutic Class:
  Antineoplastic

GENERAL USES:
Lung cancer, cervical cancer

DOSAGE FORMS:
Capsules: 0.25 mg, 1 mg; Injection: 4 mg

TOREMIFENE
tore EM i feen

TRADE NAME(S):
Fareston

THERAPEUTIC CLASS:
Antiestrogen/ antineoplastic

GENERAL USES:
Breast cancer

DOSAGE FORMS:
Tablets: 60 mg

TORSEMIDE
TORE se mide

TRADE NAME(S):
Demadex

THERAPEUTIC CLASS:
Diuretic

GENERAL USES:
CHF-related edema, hypertension

DOSAGE FORMS:
Tablets: 5 mg, 10 mg, 20 mg, 100 mg

TOSITUMOMAB/ IODINE I 131 TOSITUMOMAB
toe si TYOO mo mab

TRADE NAME(S):
Bexxar

THERAPEUTIC CLASS:
Antineoplastic

GENERAL USES:
Non-Hodgkin's lymphoma

DOSAGE FORMS:
Injection: 35 mg, 225 mg

TRAMADOL
TRA ma dole

TRADE NAME(S):
Ultram, Ultram ER, Ryzolt

THERAPEUTIC CLASS:
Analgesic

GENERAL USES:
Pain

DOSAGE FORMS:
Tablets: 50 mg; Extended-release tablets: 100 mg, 200 mg, 300 mg; Extended-release capsules: 100 mg

TRAMADOL/ ACETAMINOPHEN
TRA ma dole/a seet a MIN oh fen

TRADE NAME(S):
Ultracet

THERAPEUTIC CLASS:
Analgesic

GENERAL USES:
Short-term treatment of pain

DOSAGE FORMS:
Tablets: 37.5 mg/325 mg

TRAMETINIB DIMETHYL SULFOXIDE
tra ME ti nib dye METH il sul FOKS ide

TRADE NAME(S):
Mekinist

THERAPEUTIC CLASS:
Antineoplastic

GENERAL USES:
Melanoma

DOSAGE FORMS:
Tablets: 0.5 mg, 1 mg, 2 mg

TRANDOLAPRIL
tran DOE la pril

TRADE NAME(S):
Mavik

THERAPEUTIC CLASS:
Antihypertensive, cardiac agent

GENERAL USES:
Hypertension, CHF

DOSAGE FORMS:
Tablets: 1 mg, 2 mg, 4 mg

TRANDOLAPRIL/ VERAPAMIL
tran DOE la pril/ver AP a mil

TRADE NAME(S):
Tarka

THERAPEUTIC CLASS:
Antihypertensive/diuretic

GENERAL USES:
Hypertension

DOSAGE FORMS:
Tablets: 1 mg/240 mg, 2 mg/240 mg, 4 mg/ 240 mg

TRANEXAMIC ACID (ORAL)
TRAN ex AM ik

TRADE NAME(S):
Lysteda

THERAPEUTIC CLASS:
Hematological agent

GENERAL USES:
Menstrual bleeding

DOSAGE FORMS:
Tablets: 650 mg

TRANYLCYPROMINE
tran il SIP roe meen

TRADE NAME(S):
Parnate

THERAPEUTIC CLASS:
Antidepressant

GENERAL USES:
Depression

DOSAGE FORMS:
Tablets: 10 mg

TRASTUZUMAB
tras TOOZ oo mab

TRADE NAME(S):
Herceptin

THERAPEUTIC CLASS:
Antineoplastic

GENERAL USES:
Breast cancer

DOSAGE FORMS:
Injection: 440 mg

TRAVOPROST
TRA voe prost
Trade Name(s):
  Travatan, Izba
Therapeutic Class:
  Ocular agent
General Uses:
  Open-angle
  glaucoma, ocular
  hypertension
Dosage Forms:
  Ophthalmic solution:
  0.003%, 0.004%

TRAZODONE
TRAZ oh done
Trade Name(s):
  Trazodone, Oleptro
Therapeutic Class:
  Antidepressant
General Uses:
  Depression
Dosage Forms:
  Extended-release tablets:
  150 mg, 300 mg; Tablets
  50 mg, 100 mg

TREPROSTINIL SODIUM
tre PROST in nil
Trade Name(s):
  Remodulin, Orenitram
Therapeutic Class:
  Cardiac agent
General Uses:
  Pulmonary arterial
  hypertension
Dosage Forms:
  Extended-release tablets:

0.125 mg, 0.025 mg, 1 mg,
2.5 mg; Injection: 1 mg,
2.5 mg, 5 mg, 10 mg

TRETINOIN (TOPICAL)
TRET i noyn
Trade Name(s):
  Retin-A, Retin-A Micro
Therapeutic Class:
  Retinoid (topical)
General Uses:
  Acne vulgaris
Dosage Forms:
  Cream and Gel: 0.025%,
  0.1%; Cream: 0.05%;
  Liquid: 0.05%; Gel:
  0.01%

**TRIAMCINOLONE
(INHALED)**
trye am SIN oh lone
Trade Name(s):
  Azmacort
Therapeutic Class:
  Corticosteroid (inhaler)
General Uses:
  Asthma (chronic)
Dosage Forms:
  Inhaler: 100 mcg/
  inhalation

**TRIAMCINOLONE
(NASAL)**
trye am SIN oh lone
Trade Name(s):
  Nasacort, Nasacort
  AQ

THERAPEUTIC CLASS:
Corticosteroid (nasal)

GENERAL USES:
Allergies

DOSAGE FORMS:
Nasal spray and Inhaler:
55 mcg/spray

TRIAMCINOLONE (ORAL)
trye am SIN oh lone

TRADE NAME(S):
Kenacort, Aristocort

THERAPEUTIC CLASS:
Glucocorticoid

GENERAL USES:
Endocrine, skin, blood
disorders

DOSAGE FORMS:
Tablets: 4 mg, 8 mg;
Syrup: 4 mg/5 mL

TRIAMCINOLONE ACETONIDE
trye am SIN oh lone

TRADE NAME(S):
Aristocort, Kenalog, Flutex

THERAPEUTIC CLASS:
Corticosteroid (topical)

GENERAL USES:
Various skin conditions

DOSAGE FORMS:
Ointment and Cream:
0.025%, 0.1%, 0.5%;
Lotion: 0.025%, 0.1%

TRIAMTERENE
trye AM ter een

TRADE NAME(S):
Dyrenium

THERAPEUTIC CLASS:
Diuretic

GENERAL USES:
CHF-related edema,
hypertension

DOSAGE FORMS:
Tablets: 50 mg, 100 mg

TRIAZOLAM
trye AY zoe lam

TRADE NAME(S):
Halcion

THERAPEUTIC CLASS:
Sedative/hypnotic

GENERAL USES:
Insomnia

DOSAGE FORMS:
Tablets: 0.125 mg,
0.25 mg

TRIFLUOPERAZINE
trye floo oh PER a zeen

TRADE NAME(S):
Stelazine

THERAPEUTIC CLASS:
Antipsychotic

GENERAL USES:
Psychotic disorders,
anxiety

DOSAGE FORMS:
Tablets: 1 mg, 2 mg,
5 mg, 10 mg;
Concentrated

solution: 10 mg/mL;
Injection: 20 mg

TRIFLURIDINE
trye FLURE i deen
TRADE NAME(S):
Viroptic
THERAPEUTIC CLASS:
Ocular agent (antiviral)
GENERAL USES:
Ocular herpes infections
DOSAGE FORMS:
Ophthalmic
solution: 1%

TRIHEXYPHENIDYL
trye heks ee FEN i dil
TRADE NAME(S):
Artane
THERAPEUTIC CLASS:
Antiparkinson agent
GENERAL USES:
Parkinson's disease,
drug-induced extra-
pyramidal
disorders
DOSAGE FORMS:
Tablets: 2 mg, 5 mg;
Sustained-release
capsules: 5 mg; Elixir:
2 mg/5 mL

**TRIMETHOPRIM/
SULFAMETHOXAZOLE**
trye METH oh prim/sul fa
meth OKS a zole

TRADE NAME(S):
Bactrim, Cotrim,
Septra
THERAPEUTIC CLASS:
Anti-infective
GENERAL USES:
Bacterial infections
DOSAGE FORMS:
Tablets: 80 mg/400 mg,
160 mg/800 mg;
Suspension: 40 mg/
200 mg/5 mL; Injection:
800 mg/160 mg,
1600 mg/320 mg

TRIMIPRAMINE
trye MI pra meen
TRADE NAME(S):
Surmontil
THERAPEUTIC CLASS:
Antidepressant
GENERAL USES:
Depression
DOSAGE FORMS:
Capsules: 25 mg, 50 mg,
100 mg

TRIPTORELIN PAMOATE
trip toe REL in
TRADE NAME(S):
Trelstar Depot, Trelstar LA
THERAPEUTIC CLASS:
Antineoplastic
GENERAL USES:
Palliative treatment of
advanced prostate cancer

DOSAGE FORMS:
Injection: 3.75 mg,
11.25 mg, 22.5 mg

TROLEANDOMYCIN
troe lee an doe MYE sin
TRADE NAME(S):
TAO
THERAPEUTIC CLASS:
Anti-infective
GENERAL USES:
Bacterial infections
DOSAGE FORMS:
Capsules: 250 mg

TROSPIUM
TROSE pee um
TRADE NAME(S):
Sanctura, Sanctura XR
THERAPEUTIC CLASS:
Antispasmodic
GENERAL USES:
Overactive bladder
DOSAGE FORMS:
Tablets: 20 mg;
Extended-release
capsules: 60 mg

TRYPAN BLUE
TRYE pan
TRADE NAME(S):
Vision Blue, Membrane
Blue
THERAPEUTIC CLASS:
Ocular agent
GENERAL USES:
Cataract surgery

DOSAGE FORMS:
Ophthalmic solution:
0.06%, 0.15%

ULIPRISTAL
oo lee PRIS tal
TRADE NAME(S):
Ella
THERAPEUTIC CLASS:
Contraceptive
GENERAL USES:
Emergency contraception
DOSAGE FORMS:
Tablets: 30 mg

**UMECLIDINIUM
BROMIDE**
yoo mek li DIN ee um
TRADE NAME(S):
Incruse Ellipta
THERAPEUTIC CLASS:
Bronchodilator
GENERAL USES:
COPD
DOSAGE FORMS:
Inhalation: 62.5 mg/
inhalation

**UMECLIDINIUM
BROMIDE/VILANTEROL**
yoo mek li DIN ee um/vye
LAN ter ol
TRADE NAME(S):
Anoro Ellipta
THERAPEUTIC CLASS:
Combination
bronchodilator

GENERAL USES:
COPD

DOSAGE FORMS:
Oral inhalation: 62.5 mcg/25 mcg per double-foil blister strip

UNOPROSTONE ISOPROPYL
yoo noe PROS tone

TRADE NAME(S):
Rescula

THERAPEUTIC CLASS:
Ocular agent

GENERAL USES:
Open-angle glaucoma, ocular hypertension

DOSAGE FORMS:
Ophthalmic solution: 0.15%

URSODIOL
ur soe DYE ole

TRADE NAME(S):
Actigall, Urso

THERAPEUTIC CLASS:
Gallstone solubilizer

GENERAL USES:
Gallstones

DOSAGE FORMS:
Capsules: 300 mg; Tablets: 250 mg, 500 mg

USTEKINUMAB
US te KIN yoo mab

TRADE NAME(S):
Stelara

THERAPEUTIC CLASS:
Interleukin antagonist

GENERAL USES:
Psoriasis, psoriatic arthritis

DOSAGE FORMS:
Injection: 45 mg, 90 mg

VALACYCLOVIR
val ay SYE kloe veer

TRADE NAME(S):
Valtrex

THERAPEUTIC CLASS:
Antiviral

GENERAL USES:
Herpes, shingles, cold sores, CMV disease

DOSAGE FORMS:
Tablets: 500 mg, 1000 mg

VALGANCICLOVIR
val gan SYE kloh veer

TRADE NAME(S):
Valcyte

THERAPEUTIC CLASS:
Antiviral

GENERAL USES:
CMV retinitis in HIV patients

DOSAGE FORMS:
Oral solution: 50 mg/mL; Tablets: 450 mg

VALPROIC ACID AND DERIVATIVES
val PROE ik AS id

TRADE NAME(S):
Depakote, Depakote ER,

Depakene, Stavzor
THERAPEUTIC CLASS:
Anticonvulsant
GENERAL USES:
Seizures, bipolar
disorders, migraines
DOSAGE FORMS:
Capsules: 250 mg;
Delayed-release tablets:
125 mg, 250 mg, 500 mg;
Extended-release tablets:
250 mg, 500 mg; Sprinkle
capsules: 125 mg; Syrup:
250 mg/5 mL; Injection:
500 mg; Delayed-release
capsules: 125 mg,
250 mg, 500 mg

VALSARTAN
val SAR tan
TRADE NAME(S):
Diovan
THERAPEUTIC CLASS:
Antihypertensive
GENERAL USES:
Hypertension, CHF
DOSAGE FORMS:
Capsules: 80 mg, 160 mg,
320 mg

VALSARTAN/HCTZ
val SAR tan/hye droe klor oh
THYE a zide
TRADE NAME(S):
Diovan HCT
THERAPEUTIC CLASS:
Antihypertensive/
diuretic

GENERAL USES:
Hypertension
DOSAGE FORMS:
Tablets: 80 mg/12.5 mg,
160 mg/12.5 mg,
320 mg/12.5 mg,
320 mg/25 mg

VANCOMYCIN
van koe MYE sin
TRADE NAME(S):
Vancocin, Vancoled
THERAPEUTIC CLASS:
Anti-infective
GENERAL USES:
Bacterial infections
DOSAGE FORMS:
Capsules: 125 mg,
250 mg; Solution: 1 g,
10 g; Injection: 500 mg,
1 g, 2 g, 5 g, 10 g

VANDETANIB
van DET a nib
TRADE NAME(S):
Caprelsa
THERAPEUTIC CLASS:
Antineoplastic
GENERAL USES:
Thyroid cancer
DOSAGE FORMS:
Tablets: 100 mg, 300 mg

VARDENAFIL
var DEN a fil
TRADE NAME(S):
Levitra, Staxyn

Therapeutic Class:
Impotence agent
General Uses:
Erectile dysfunction
Dosage Forms:
Tablets: 2.5 mg, 5 mg, 10 mg, 20 mg; Orally disintegrating tablets: 10 mg

VARENICLINE
var e NI kleen
Trade Name(s):
Chantix
Therapeutic Class:
Nicotine agonist
General Uses:
Smoking cessation
Dosage Forms:
Tablets: 0.5 mg, 1 mg

VARICELLA VACCINE
var ih SELL ah
Trade Name(s):
Varivax
Therapeutic Class:
Vaccine
General Uses:
Prevention of chickenpox
Dosage Forms:
Injection: 0.5 mL

VECURONIUM
ve kyoo ROE ni um
Trade Name(s):
Norcuron
Therapeutic Class:
Muscle relaxant

General Uses:
Aid to anesthesia
Dosage Forms:
Injection: 10 mg, 20 mg

VEDOLIZUMAB
VE doe LIZ oo mab
Trade Name(s):
Entyvio
Therapeutic Class:
Antibody
General Uses:
Ulcerative colitis, Crohn's disease
Dosage Forms:
Injection: 300 mg

VELAGLUCERASE ALFA
VEL a GLOO ser ase
Trade Name(s):
Vpriv
Therapeutic Class:
Enzyme
General Uses:
Gaucher's disease (type 1)
Dosage Forms:
Injection: 200 units, 400 units

VEMURAFENIB
VEM yoo RAF e nib
Trade Name(s):
Zelboraf
Therapeutic Class:
Antineoplastic
General Uses:
Metastatic melanoma

DOSAGE FORMS:
Tablets: 240 mg

VENLAFAXINE
ven la FAKS een
TRADE NAME(S):
Effexor, Effexor XR
THERAPEUTIC CLASS:
Antidepressant
GENERAL USES:
Depression, social anxiety
disorder, panic disorder
DOSAGE FORMS:
Tablets: 25 mg, 37.5 mg,
50 mg, 75 mg, 100 mg;
Extended-release tablets:
37.5 mg, 75 mg, 150 mg

VERAPAMIL
ver AP a mil
TRADE NAME(S):
Calan, Isoptin, Verelan,
Isoptin SR, Calan SR,
Verelan PM
THERAPEUTIC CLASS:
Antihypertensive (SR),
antianginal
GENERAL USES:
Hypertension, angina
DOSAGE FORMS:
Tablets: 40 mg, 80 mg,
120 mg; Sustained-
release tablets and
Capsules: 120 mg,
180 mg, 240 mg;
Sustained-release
capsules: 100 mg,

200 mg, 300 mg;
Injection: 5 mg

VIDARABINE
vye DARE a been
TRADE NAME(S):
Vira-A
THERAPEUTIC CLASS:
Ocular agent (antiviral)
GENERAL USES:
Ocular herpes
infections
DOSAGE FORMS:
Ophthalmic ointment: 3%

VIGABATRIN
vye GA ba trin
TRADE NAME(S):
Sabril
THERAPEUTIC CLASS:
Anticonvulsant
GENERAL USES:
Seizures
DOSAGE FORMS:
Tablets: 500 mg; Solution:
500 mg

VILAZODONE HCL
vil AZ oh done
TRADE NAME(S):
Viibryd
THERAPEUTIC CLASS:
Antidepressant
GENERAL USES:
Depression
DOSAGE FORMS:
Tablets: 10 mg, 20 mg,
40 mg

VINBLASTINE
vin BLAS teen

TRADE NAME(S):
Velban

THERAPEUTIC CLASS:
Antineoplastic

GENERAL USES:
Various cancers

DOSAGE FORMS:
Injection: 10 mg,
25 mg

VINCRISTINE
vin KRIS teen

TRADE NAME(S):
Vincasar PFS

THERAPEUTIC CLASS:
Antineoplastic

GENERAL USES:
Various cancers

DOSAGE FORMS:
Injection: 1 mg, 2 mg,
5 mg

VINCRISTINE SULFATE (LIPOSOMAL)
vin KRIS teen

TRADE NAME(S):
Marqibo

THERAPEUTIC CLASS:
Antineoplastic

GENERAL USES:
ALL

DOSAGE FORMS:
Injection: 5 mg

VINORELBINE
vi NOR el been

TRADE NAME(S):
Navelbine

THERAPEUTIC CLASS:
Antineoplastic

GENERAL USES:
Various cancers

DOSAGE FORMS:
Injection: 10 mg, 50 mg

VISMODEGIB
VIS moe DEG ib

TRADE NAME(S):
Erivedge

THERAPEUTIC CLASS:
Antineoplastic

GENERAL USES:
Metastatic basal cell
cancer

DOSAGE FORMS:
Capsules: 150 mg

VITAMIN K (PHYTONADIONE)
fye toe na DYE one

TRADE NAME(S):
Aqua-Mephyton,
Mephyton

THERAPEUTIC CLASS:
Vitamin

GENERAL USES:
Blood-clotting
disorders

DOSAGE FORMS:
Tablets: 5 mg; Injection:
1 mg

VORAPAXAR
VOR a PAX ar
TRADE NAME(S):
Zontivity
THERAPEUTIC CLASS:
Antiplatelet agent
GENERAL USES:
Reduce stroke, MI risk, and acute coronary syndrome
DOSAGE FORMS:
Tablets: 2.08 mg

VORICONAZOLE
vor i KOE na zole
TRADE NAME(S):
VFEND
THERAPEUTIC CLASS:
Antifungal
GENERAL USES:
Serious fungal infections
DOSAGE FORMS:
Tablets: 50 mg, 200 mg; Injection: 200 mg

VORINOSTAT
vor IN oh stat
TRADE NAME(S):
Zolinza
THERAPEUTIC CLASS:
Enzyme inhibitor
GENERAL USES:
Cutaneous T-cell lymphoma
DOSAGE FORMS:
Capsules: 100 mg

VORTIOXETINE
VOR tye OKS e teen
TRADE NAME(S):
Brintellix
THERAPEUTIC CLASS:
Antidepressant
GENERAL USES:
Depression
DOSAGE FORMS:
Tablets: 5 mg, 10 mg, 15 mg, 20 mg

WARFARIN
WAR far in
TRADE NAME(S):
Coumadin
THERAPEUTIC CLASS:
Anticoagulant
GENERAL USES:
Prevent blood clots
DOSAGE FORMS:
Tablets: 1 mg, 2 mg, 2.5 mg, 3 mg, 4 mg, 5 mg, 6 mg, 7.5 mg, 10 mg

ZAFIRLUKAST
za FIR loo kast
TRADE NAME(S):
Accolate
THERAPEUTIC CLASS:
Bronchodilator
GENERAL USES:
Asthma prevention and treatment
DOSAGE FORMS:
Tablets: 10 mg, 20 mg

ZALEPLON
ZAL e plon
TRADE NAME(S):
Sonata
THERAPEUTIC CLASS:
Hypnotic/sedative
GENERAL USES:
Insomnia
DOSAGE FORMS:
Capsules: 5 mg,
10 mg

ZANAMIVIR
za NA mi veer
TRADE NAME(S):
Relenza
THERAPEUTIC CLASS:
Antiviral
GENERAL USES:
Influenza A and B
DOSAGE FORMS:
Inhalation: 5 mg/
inhalation

ZICONOTIDE
zi KOE no tide
TRADE NAME(S):
Prialt
THERAPEUTIC CLASS:
Analgesic
GENERAL USES:
Severe chronic pain
DOSAGE FORMS:
Injection: 100 mcg,
200 mcg, 500 mcg

ZIDOVUDINE
zye DOE vyoo deen
TRADE NAME(S):
Retrovir
THERAPEUTIC CLASS:
Antiviral
GENERAL USES:
HIV infection
DOSAGE FORMS:
Capsules: 100 mg;
Tablets: 300 mg; Syrup:
50 mg/mL; Injection:
200 mg

ZILEUTON
zye LOO ton
TRADE NAME(S):
Zyflo CR
THERAPEUTIC CLASS:
Antiasthmatic
GENERAL USES:
Asthma prevention and
treatment
DOSAGE FORMS:
Extended-release tablets:
600 mg

ZIPRASIDONE
zi PRAS i done
TRADE NAME(S):
Geodon
THERAPEUTIC CLASS:
Antipsychotic
GENERAL USES:
Schizophrenia, bipolar
mania

DOSAGE FORMS:
Capsules: 20 mg, 40 mg, 60 mg, 80 mg; Injection: 20 mg

ZIV-AFLIBERCEPT
ziv a FLIH ber sept
TRADE NAME(S):
Zaltrap
THERAPEUTIC CLASS:
Antineoplastic
GENERAL USES:
Metastatic colorectal cancer
DOSAGE FORMS:
Injection: 100 mg, 200 mg

ZOLEDRONIC ACID
zoe le DRON ik AS id
TRADE NAME(S):
Zometa, Reclast
THERAPEUTIC CLASS:
Bisphosphonate
GENERAL USES:
Hypercalcemia related to cancer, osteoporosis, Paget's disease
DOSAGE FORMS:
Injection: 4 mg, 5 mg

ZOLMITRIPTAN
zohl mi TRIP tan
TRADE NAME(S):
Zomig, Zomig-ZMT
THERAPEUTIC CLASS:
Antimigraine

GENERAL USES:
Migraines
DOSAGE FORMS:
Tablets: 2.5 mg, 5 mg; Orally disintegrating tablets: 2.5 mg, 5 mg; Nasal spray: 5 mg/0.1 mL

ZOLPIDEM
zole PI dem
TRADE NAME(S):
Ambien, Ambien CR, Edular, Zolpimist
THERAPEUTIC CLASS:
Sedative, hypnotic
GENERAL USES:
Insomnia
DOSAGE FORMS:
Sublingual tablets and Tablets: 5 mg, 10 mg; Extended-release tablets: 6.25 mg, 12.5 mg; Spray (oral): 5 mg/spray

ZONISAMIDE
zoe NIS a mide
TRADE NAME(S):
Zonegran
THERAPEUTIC CLASS:
Anticonvulsant
GENERAL USES:
Partial seizures (adults)
DOSAGE FORMS:
Capsules: 25 mg, 50 mg, 100 mg

ZOSTER VACCINE
ZOS ter vak SEEN

TRADE NAME(S):
Zostavax

THERAPEUTIC CLASS:
Vaccine

GENERAL USES:
Prevent herpes
zoster (shingles)

DOSAGE FORMS:
Injection: 0.65 mL

Appendix A: Top 200 Drugs (Selected From Community and Hospital Settings)

Generic Name	Brand Name	General Use(s)
Abacavir/lamivudine	Epzicom	HIV infection
Adalimumab	Humira	Rheumatoid arthritis, ankylosing spondylitis, inflammatory bowel disease
Albuterol (aerosol)	Proventil HFA, ProAir HFA, Ventolin HFA	Bronchospasm
Alendronate	Fosamax	Osteoporosis, Paget's disease
Alprazolam	Xanax	Anxiety, panic disorder
Amlodipine	Norvasc	Angina, hypertension
Amlodipine/valsartan	Exforge	Hypertension
Amoxicillin	Amoxicot, Amoxil, Moxatag, Moxilin, Trimox	Bacterial infections
Aripiprazole	Abilify	Psychotic disorders
Aspirin/dipyridamole	Aggrenox	Reduce stroke risk
Atazanavir	Reyataz	HIV Infection

Top 200 Drugs (CONTINUED)

Atomoxetine	Strattera	ADHD
Atorvastatin	Lipitor	Hyperlipidemia, hypertriglyceridemia, reduce stroke or MI risk
Azelastine (nasal spray)	Astelin	Seasonal allergies
Azithromycin	Zithromax	Bacterial infections
Beclomethasone (inhaled)	Qvar	Asthma (chronic)
Bevacizumab	Avastin	Metastatic colorectal cancer
Bimatoprost (ophthalmic solution)	Lumigan, Latisse	Ocular hypertension, open-angle glaucoma, promote eyelash growth
Bivalirudin	Angiomax	Prevent clotting in angina/PTCA
Brimonidine (ophthalmic solution)	Alphagan P	Glaucoma, ocular hypertension
Budesonide (nasal spray)	Rhinocort Aqua	Allergies
Budesonide/formoterol	Symbicort	Asthma, COPD
Buprenorphine/naloxone	Suboxone	Opioid dependence
Bupropion (extended/sustained release)	Wellbutrin XL, Budeprion SR	Depression, seasonal affective disorder

Capecitabine	Xeloda	Metastatic breast cancer
Carvedilol	Coreg	Hypertension, CHF
Ceftriaxone	Rocephin	Bacterial infections
Celecoxib	Celebrex	Osteoarthritis, rheumatoid arthritis, acute pain, dysmenorrhea, FAP
Cephalexin	Keflex	Bacterial infections
Cetuximab	Erbitux	Various cancers
Cinacalcet	Sensipar	Secondary hyperparathyroidism, hypercalcemia in parathyroid cancer
Ciprofloxacin/dexamethasone (otic)	Ciprodex	Acute otitis media
Citalopram	Celexa	Depression
Clopidogrel	Plavix	Reduce stroke, MI risk, acute coronary syndrome
Colchicine	Colcrys	Gout, familial Mediterranean fever
Cyclosporine (ocular)	Restasis	Increase tear production
Dabigatran etexilate mesylate	Pradaxa	Reduce risk of stroke, prevent and treat clots

Top 200 Drugs (continued)

Dalteparin sodium	Fragmin	Prevent blood clots
Daptomycin	Cubicin	Bacterial infections
Darbepoetin alfa	Aranesp	Anemia
Darunavir	Prezista	HIV infection
Desvenlafaxine	Pristiq	Depression
Dexmethylphenidate	Focalin XR	ADHD
Dextroamphetamine/amphetamine	Adderall, Adderall XR	ADHD
Diclofenac (gel)	Voltaren Gel	Osteoarthritis (knee, hand)
Digoxin	Digitek, Lanoxin	CHF, atrial fibrillation
Diltiazem	Cardizem, Tiazac	Hypertension, angina
Donepezil	Aricept	Alzheimer's disease
Dorzolamide/timolol	Cosopt	Glaucoma, ocular hypertension
Doxycycline	Atridox, Alodox, Vibramycin	Bacterial infection
Duloxetine	Cymbalta	Anxiety, depression, fibromyalgia
Dutasteride	Avodart	BPH

Efavirenz/emtricitabine/tenofovir	Atripla	HIV infection
Eletriptan	Relpax	Migraines
Enoxaparin sodium	Lovenox	Prevent blood clots
Epoetin alfa	Epogen, Procrit	Anemia with chronic renal failure, cancer, HIV infection
Escitalopram	Lexapro	Depression, anxiety
Esomeprazole	Nexium	GERD, erosive esophagitis, Zollinger-Ellison syndrome, decrease risk of NSAID associated ulcer
Estradiol (transdermal)	Vivelle-Dot, Climara	Estrogen replacement
Estrogens, conjugated/ medroxyprogesterone	Prempro	Estrogen replacement
Estrogens, conjugated	Premarin, Cenestin	Estrogen replacement
Eszopiclone	Lunesta	Insomnia
Etanercet	Enbrel	Rheumatoid and psoriatic arthritis, plaque psoriasis, ankylosing spondylitis
Ethinyl estradiol/desogestrel	Apri, Mircette, Kariva	Contraception

Top 200 Drugs (continued)

Ethinyl estradiol/drospirenone	Yasmin, Yaz	Contraception
Ethinyl estradiol/ethynodiol	Zovia 1/35e	Contraception
Ethinyl estradiol/etonogestrel	NuvaRing	Contraception
Ethinyl estradiol/levonorgestrel	Aviane, Alesse	Contraception
Ethinyl estradiol/norethindrone/ ferrous fumarate	Loestrin 24 Fe, Microgestin, Minastrin 24 Fe	Contraception
Ethinyl estradiol/norgestimate	Sprintec, Ortho-Cyclen, Ortho-Tri-Cyclen	Contraception
Exenatide	Byetta	Diabetes (type 2)
Ezetimibe	Zetia	Hyperlipidemia
Ezetimibe/simvastatin	Vytorin	Hypercholesterolemia
Fenofibrate	TriCor	Hyperlipidemia
Fenofibric acid	Trilipix	Hyperlipidemia
Fentanyl	Fentanyl	Pain
Finasteride	Proscar, Propecia	BPH, male-pattern baldness

Fluoxetine	Prozac	Depression, bulimia, OCD, PMDD
Fluticasone (inhaler)	Flovent HFA	Asthma (chronic)
Fluticasone (nasal)	Veramyst	Allergies
Fluticasone/salmeterol	Advair Diskus	Asthma (chronic), COPD
Furosemide	Lasix	CHF- and pulmonary-related edema, hypertension
Gabapentin	Neurontin	Seizures, postherpetic neuralgia
Glatiramer acetate	Copaxone	Multiple sclerosis
Glimepiride	Amaryl	Diabetes (type 2)
Hydrochlorothiazide	Microzide	Diuretic
Hydrocodone/acetaminophen	Lorcet, Lortab, Norco, Vicodin	Pain
Ibandronate	Boniva	Postmenopausal osteoporosis
Imatinib	Gleevec	CML, GI stromal tumors, ALL
Infliximab	Remicade	Crohn's disease, various arthritis syndromes, ulcerative colitis, psoriasis, psoriatic arthritis

Top 200 Drugs (continued)

Insulin, aspart	Novolog	Diabetes
Insulin, detemir	Levemir	Diabetes
Insulin, glargine	Lantus, Lantus SoloSTAR	Diabetes
Insulin, lispro	Humalog	Diabetes
Ipilimumab	Yervoy	Metastatic melanoma
Ipratropium/albuterol (inhaler)	Combivent Respimat	Bronchospasm
Irbesartan	Avapro	Hypertension, diabetic nephropathy
Lamotrigine	Lamictal	Seizures, bipolar disorder
Lansoprazole	Prevacid	GERD, duodenal ulcer
Latanoprost (ophthalmic solution)	Xalatan	Glaucoma, ocular hypertension
Levalbuterol (inhalation)	Xopenex	Bronchospasm
Levetiracetam	Keppra	Seizures
Levofloxacin	Levaquin	Bacterial infections
Levothyroxine	Synthroid, Levoxyl, Levothroid	Hypothyroidism

TOP 200 DRUGS (CONTINUED)

Lidocaine (transdermal)	Lidoderm	Postherpetic neuralgia
Linezolid	Zyvox	Vancomycin-resistant bacterial infections
Liraglutide	Victoza	Diabetes (type 2)
Lisdexamfetamine dimesylate	Vyvanse	ADHD
Lisinopril	Prinivil, Zestril	Hypertension, heart failure, MI
Losartan	Cozaar	Hypertension, diabetic nephropathy
Losartan/HCTZ	Hyzaar	Antihypertensive/diuretic
Memantine	Namenda	Alzheimer's disease
Mesalamine	Asacol, Lialda	Inflammatory bowel disease
Metformin	Fortamet, Glucophage	Diabetes (type 2)
Methotrexate	Rheumatrex, Trexall	Cancer, rheumatoid arthritis, psoriasis
Methylphenidate	Concerta, Methylin	ADHD, narcolepsy
Metoprolol (extended-release)	Toprol XL	Hypertension, angina, MI
Metronidazole	Flagyl	Bacterial infections, gastric ulcers
Minocycline	Solodyn	Bacterial infections, acne

Modafinil	Provigil	Narcolepsy, fatigue associated with sleep apnea and sleep disorders
Mometasone (nasal)	Nasonex	Allergies
Montelukast	Singulair	Asthma prevention and treatment, seasonal allergies
Morphine sulfate	Morphine sulfate	Pain
Moxifloxacin	Avelox	Bacterial infections
Mupirocin (topical)	Bactroban	Impetigo, skin infection
Niacin	Niaspan	Hyperlipidemia
Nitroglycerin (sublingual)	NitroQuick, Nitrostat, Nitrolingual	Angina
Olanzapine	Zyprexa	Psychotic disorders
Olmesartan	Benicar	Hypertension
Olmesartan/HCTZ	Benicar HCT	Antihypertensive/diuretic
Olopatadine (ophthalmic solution)	Patanol	Allergic conjunctivitis
Omalizumab	Xolair	Asthma, chronic idiopathic urticaria

TOP 200 DRUGS (CONTINUED)

Omega-3 acid ethyl esters	Lovaza	Hypertriglyceridemia
Omeprazole	Prilosec	GERD, duodenal ulcer
Oxaliplatin	Eloxatin	Colon or rectal cancer (metastatic)
Oxcarbazepine	Trileptal	Partial seizures
Oxycodone	OxyContin, Roxicodone	Pain
Oxycodone/acetaminophen	Endocet, Percocet, Roxicet	Pain
Oxymorphone	Opana ER	Pain
Paclitaxel	Taxol	Various cancers
Palonosetron	Aloxi	Chemotherapy-induced nausea/vomiting
Pantoprazole	Protonix	GERD, erosive esophagitis
Paroxetine (controlled release)	Paxil CR	Depression, OCD, panic disorder, social anxiety, PMDD, PTSD, menopause
Pegfilgrastim	Neulasta	Prevent infection in cancer patients
Pioglitazone	Actos	Diabetes (type 2)
Piperacillin/tazobactam	Zosyn	Bacterial infections

Potassium chloride	Klor-Con	Potassium replacement
Pravastatin	Pravachol	Hyperlipidemia
Pregabalin	Lyrica	Seizures, fibromyalgia, neuropathic pain
Quetiapine	Seroquel	Psychotic disorders
Rabeprazole	Aciphex	GERD, duodenal ulcer, hyperacidity disorders
Raloxifene	Evista	Osteoporosis prevention, breast cancer
Raltegravir	Isentress	HIV Infection
Ramipril	Altace	Hypertension, heart failure
Ranibizumab	Lucentis	Wet macular degeneration, diabetic macular edema
Ranolazine	Ranexa	Chronic angina
Rifaximin	Xifaxan	Traveler's diarrhea, hepatic encephalopathy
Risedronate	Actonel	Osteoporosis, Paget's disease
Risperidone	Risperdal	Psychotic disorders
Rituximab	Rituxan	Rheumatoid arthritis, non-Hodgkin's lymphoma
Rivaroxaban	Xarelto	Treat and prevent blood clots

Rivastigmine (transdermal)	Exelon	Alzheimer's disease, Parkinson's dementia
Rizatriptan	Maxalt, Maxalt-MLT	Migraines
Ropinirole	Requip, Requip XL	Parkinson's disease, restless leg syndrome
Rosuvastatin	Crestor	Hyperlipidemia
Salmeterol (inhalation)	Serevent Diskus	Asthma, COPD, bronchospasm
Saxagliptin	Onglyza	Diabetes (type 2)
Sertraline	Zoloft	Depression, social anxiety disorder, OCD, PMDD, panic disorder
Sildenafil	Viagra	Erectile dysfunction
Simvastatin	Zocor	Hyperlipidemia, CHD
Sitagliptin	Januvia	Diabetes (type 2)
Sitagliptin/metformin	Janumet	Diabetes (type 2)
Solifenacin succinate	VESIcare	Overactive bladder
Tacrolimus	Prograf	Prevent organ transplant rejection
Tadalafil	Cialis	Erectile dysfunction, PAH, BPH

Top 200 Drugs (continued)

Tamsulosin	Flomax	BPH
Telaprevir	Incivek	Chronic hepatitis C
Tenofovir	Viread	HIV Infection
Tenofovir/emtricitabine	Truvada	HIV infection
Teriparatide	Forteo	Postmenopausal osteoporosis
Testosterone (topical)	Androgel	Replacement therapy (men)
Tiotropium bromide	Spiriva	COPD
Tolderodine (long acting)	Detrol LA	Bladder instability
Topiramate	Topamax	Seizures, migraines
Tramadol	Ultram ER, Ultram	Pain
Trastuzumab	Herceptin	Breast cancer
Travoprost (ocular)	Travatan Z	Open-angle glaucoma, ocular hypertension
Triamcinolone (nasal spray)	Nasacort AQ	Allergies
Valganciclovir	Valcyte	CMV retinitis in HIV patients
Valproic acid (extended release)	Depakote, Depakote ER	Seizures, bipolar disorder, migraines

Top 200 Drugs (continued)

Valsartan	Diovan	Hypertension, CHF
Valsartan/HCTZ	Diovan HCT	Hypertension
Vardenafil	Levitra	Erectile dysfunction
Varenicline	Chantix	Smoking cessation
Venlafaxine (extended release)	Effexor XR	Depression, social anxiety disorder, panic disorder
Warfarin	Coumadin	Prevent blood clots
Ziprasidone	Geodon	Schizophrenia, bipolar mania
Zoledronic acid	Reclast, Zometa	Hypercalcemia related to cancer, osteoporosis, Paget's disease
Zolpidem	Ambien, Ambien CR	Insomnia
Zoster vaccine	Zostavax	Prevent herpes zoster (shingles)

The Drug Enforcement Administration (DEA) has the authority to specify which drugs need special controls. These drugs are defined in five categories of controlled substances:

- *Schedule I* drugs have high abuse and addiction potential and have no accepted medical use in the United States. Examples include heroin, LSD, marijuana, mescaline, 3,4-methylenedioxymethamphetamine ("Ecstasy"), and psilocin ("mushrooms").
- *Schedule II* drugs have high abuse and addiction potential but do have medical applications. Examples include cocaine, Dilaudid (hydromorphone), Ritalin (methylphenidate), Seconal (secobarbital), MS Contin (morphine), various opiate analgesics, and several types of amphetamines ("diet pills" or "speed").
- *Schedule III* drugs have abuse and addiction potential but not as much as those in Schedule II. Examples include Tylenol #3 (acetaminophen with codeine), Fastin (phentermine), anabolic steroids, and Marinol (THC).
- *Schedule IV* drugs have a low potential for abuse. Examples include Valium (diazepam), Halcion (triazolam), Somnote (chloral hydrate), Ambien (zolpidem), and Versed (midazolam).
- *Schedule V* drugs have low abuse potential and have very limited amounts of drugs in each dosage form. Examples are Lomotil (diphenoxylate and atropine) and some cough syrups containing codeine. Some Schedule V products do not even require a prescription (because of FDA regulations), but they must be dispensed by a pharmacist because of DEA rules.

Source: Posey LM. *Complete Review for the Pharmacy Technician,* 2nd edition. Washington, DC: American Pharmacists Association; 2007. Adapted with permission.

$\bar{a}$	before
$\overline{aa}$	of each
a.c.	before meals
ad	up to
A.D.	right ear
ad lib	at pleasure
a.m.	morning
ante	before
aq	aqueous (water)
A.S.	left ear
A.U.	each ear or both ears
b.i.d.	twice a day
$\bar{c}$	with
cap	capsule
cc	cubic centimeter (milliliter)
Cl	chloride
comp	compound
D.A.W.	dispense as written
D.C., dc, or disc	discontinue
dil	dilute
disp	dispense
div	divide
dx	diagnosis
D5NS	5% dextrose in 0.9% sodium chloride
D5RL	5% dextrose in Ringer's lactate
D5W	5% dextrose in water
elix	elixir
et	and
ft	make
g	gram
gal	gallon
gr	grain
gtt	drop
h or hr	hour
h.s.	at bedtime

hx	history
H_2O	water
IM	intramuscular
inj	injection
IV	intravenous
IVP	intravenous push
IVPB	intravenous piggyback
K	potassium
KCl	potassium chloride
L or l	liter
lb	pound
LR	lactated Ringer's
MBq	megabecquerel
mcg or μg	microgram
mCi	millicurie
mEq	milliequivalent
Mg	magnesium
mg	milligram
min	minute
mL or ml	milliliter
Na	sodium
NaCl	sodium chloride
N.F.	National Formulary
noct	night
non rep	do not repeat
NPO	nothing by mouth
NR	no refill
NS	normal saline (0.9% sodium chloride)
NTG	nitroglycerin
N/V	nausea and/or vomiting
O.D.	right eye
O.S. or O.L.	left eye
O.U.	each eye or both eyes
oz	ounce
$\bar{p}$	after
p.c.	after meals
p.m.	afternoon; evening

p.o. or PO	by mouth
PR	per rectum
p.r.n.	as needed
pt	pint
pulv	powder
q	every
q.d.	every day
q.h.	every hour
q.h.s.	every bedtime
q.i.d.	four times a day
q.o.d.	every other day
q.s. or qs	a sufficient quantity
q.s. ad	a sufficient quantity to make
qt	quart
RL	Ringer's lactate
R/O	rule out
$\bar{s}$	without
sec	second
Sig.	write on label
SL, sl	sublingual
sol	solution
$\overline{ss}$	one half
SSKI	saturated solution of potassium iodide
stat	immediately
s.c. or s.q.	subcutaneously
supp	suppository
susp	suspension
syr	syrup
tab.	tablet
tbsp or T	tablespoonful
t.i.d.	three times a day
TPN	total parenteral nutrition
tr or tinct	tincture
tsp or t	teaspoonful
ung	ointment
U.S.P.	United States Pharmacopeia

Temperature

Fahrenheit to Centigrade or Celsius: $(°F - 32) \times 5/9 = °C$
Centigrade or Celsius to Fahrenheit: $(°C \times 9/5) + 32 = °F$

°C	=	°F	°C	=	°F	°C	=	°F
100.0		212.0	39.0		102.2	36.8		98.2
50.0		122.0	38.8		101.8	36.6		97.9
41.0		105.8	38.6		101.5	36.4		97.5
40.8		105.4	38.4		101.1	36.2		97.2
40.6		105.1	38.2		100.8	36.0		96.8
40.4		104.7	38.0		100.4	35.8		96.4
40.2		104.4	37.8		100.1	35.6		96.1
40.0		104.0	37.6		99.7	35.4		95.7
39.8		103.6	37.4		99.3	35.2		95.4
39.6		103.3	37.2		99.0	35.5		95.0
39.4		102.9	37.0		98.6	0		32.0
39.2		102.6						

Pounds to Kilograms

lb	=	kg	lb	=	kg	lb	=	kg
1		0.45	70		31.75	140		63.50
5		2.27	75		34.02	145		65.77
10		4.54	80		36.29	150		68.04
15		6.80	85		38.56	155		70.31
20		9.07	90		40.82	160		72.58
25		11.34	95		43.09	165		74.84
30		13.61	100		45.36	170		77.11
35		15.88	105		47.63	175		79.38
40		18.14	110		49.90	180		81.65
45		20.41	115		52.16	185		83.92
50		22.68	120		54.43	190		86.18
55		24.95	125		56.70	195		88.45
60		27.22	130		58.91	200		90.72
65		29.48	135		61.24			

Exact Equivalents

1 oz	=	28.35 g
1 lb	=	453.6 g (0.4536 kg)
1 kg	=	2.2 lb
1 fluid oz (fl oz)	=	29.57 mL
1 pint (pt)	=	473.2 mL
1 quart (qt)	=	946.4 mL

Metric Conversions

1 kg	=	1000 g
1 g	=	1000 mg
1 mg	=	1000 mcg or μg

Approximate Measures: Liquids

1 fl oz	=	30 mL
1 cup (8 fl oz)	=	240 mL
1 pint (16 fl oz)	=	480 mL
1 quart (32 fl oz)	=	960 mL
1 gallon (128 fl oz)	=	3800 mL
1 teaspoon	=	5 mL
1 tablespoon	=	15 mL

Approximate Measures: Weights

1 oz	=	30 g
1 lb (16 oz)	=	480 g
15 grains	=	1 g
1 grain	=	60 mg

P

Q

QNASL (beclomethasone), 23
Qsymia (phentermine/
    topiramate), 181
Quaexy XR (topiramate), 221
Quartette (ethinyl estradiol/
    levonorgestrel), 87
Quillivant XR
    (methylphenidate), 147
Quinaglute (quinidine
    gluconate), 191
Quinalan (quinidine gluconate),
    191
Quinaretic (quinapril/HCTZ),
    191
Quinidex Extentabs (quinidine
    sulfate), 191
Quinine (quinine sulfate), 191
Quinora (quinidine sulfate), 191
Qutenza (capsaicin,
    transdermal), 36
Qvar (beclomethasone,
    inhaled), 23

R

Raguro (methotrexate), 146
Ranexa (ranolazine), 193
Rapaflo (silodosin), 203
Rapamune (sirolimus), 204
Raptiva (efalizumab), 72
Ravicti (glycerol
    phenylbutyrate), 109
Raxibacumab (raxibacumab),
    193

Rayos (prednisone), 187
Razadyne (galantamine), 106
Rebetrol (ribavirin, oral), 195
Rebif (interferon beta-1a), 122
Reclast (zoledronic acid), 235
Reclomide (metoclopramide),
    148
Rectiv (nitroglycerin, rectal),
    162
Refludan (lepirudin), 131
Reglan (metoclopramide), 148
Regranex (becaplermin), 23
Relafen (nabumetone), 156
Relenza (zanamivir), 234
Relistor (methylnaltrexone), 147
Relpax (eletriptan), 73
Remeron (mirtazapine), 153
Remicade (infliximab), 119
Remodulin (treprostinil
    sodium), 224
Remular (chlorzoxazone), 46
Renagel (sevelamer
    hydrochloride), 203
Renvela (sevelamer carbonate),
    202
Reprexain (hydrocodone/
    ibuprofen), 114
Requip (ropinirole), 199
Rescriptor (delavirdine), 59
Rescula (unoprostone
    isopropyl), 228
Restasis (cyclosporine, ocular),
    56
Restoril (temazepam), 212
Retavase (reteplase), 194